super
feast

michael van straten

recipes by sally van straten

super feast

First published in the United Kingdom in 2005 by Little Books Ltd,
48 Catherine Place, London SW1E 6HL

10 9 8 7 6 5 4 3 2 1

A CIP catalogue record for this book is available from the British Library.

ISBN: 1 904435 41 6

Many thanks to: Jamie Ambrose for editorial production and management,
Ann Barrett for indexing,
Claudia Dowell for proofreading,
Debbie Clement for jacket design,
Mousemat Design Limited for text design.
Printed and bound by CTP Printing in Hong Kong

contents

introduction

how to use this book

Some people eat to live, some live to eat, but a combination of both is by far the happiest and healthiest path to follow. Food is pleasure – and I'm not just talking about how it looks, smells or tastes. Tragically, the far more subtle social pleasures of eating together with friends and family are a rare occurrence in today's 24/7 society. It's sitting around the table that gives children their earliest introduction to social intercourse, the enjoyment of eating and the development of a complex palate which can savour a multitude of flavours. Now is the time to turn back the clock and rebel against the fast-food, junk-food and synthetic-food industry. This is how to stem the tide of rising childhood obesity, the ever-increasing toll of diabetic children and premature deaths from heart disease, strokes and many forms of cancer.

Writing this book has been a bit like *Desert Island Discs* – choosing the eight records is not so hard; it's leaving out all the others that's the most difficult. With only room for one hundred foods, what did I leave out? That is a question I spent many hours agonizing over. Yet here is a distillation of the best hundred foods in the world. This is not a diet book, a nutrition book, or a health book. It is an *eating* book.

The first way to use this book is as a simple and practical guide to everyday shopping, cooking and eating. Do this and you'll always have a super-abundance of essential vitamins and minerals. Just as importantly, you'll achieve an intake of the thousands of natural plant chemicals (phytochemicals) – most of which you can't get from pills and many of which have yet to be identified – that help protect every single cell in your body.

You can also use this book to increase your consumption of specific nutrients your body may need more of from time to time. For example, you may be entering a period of extra stress: exams, new job, moving house, marriage, divorce. It's at this time that you need extra B vitamins for your central nervous system, feel-good phytochemicals from specific foods, herbs and spices, or Nature's ingredients to help you get a good night's sleep. You'll find recipes and menu suggestions in the section on beating stress.

If there's a 'flu epidemic, everyone around you is catching colds, or you're waiting to go into hospital for that long-planned hip replacement, now's the time to eat from the 'protective' section to boost your natural immunity. Maybe you've been overindulging a little and piled on a few pounds. Simply turn to the 'low-carb' section and eat your fill of balanced, satisfying, but reduced-calorie dishes and watch the weight vanish.

In the recipe sections, you'll also find meals to boost vitality, food and drink for an instant pick-me-up, and suggestions for cleansing your system – including a great three-day detox diet I've used for my patients for many years. There is even an aphrodisiac section that contains recipes to enchant your partner on Valentine's Day or any other romantic occasion.

Finally, at the end of the book you'll find the 'supercures' section, which follows the words of Hippocrates, the father of modern medicine: 'Let food be your medicine and let medicine be your food.' This section isn't a substitute for professional health advice, but a simple guide to using food as first-aid in the relief of many ailments, from acne to chronic fatigue, arthritis to depression, headaches and heart disease to PMS, prostate problems and varicose veins.

When I qualified in 1964, naturopaths like me were seen as cranks by the scientific and medical establishments. I was accused of being a charlatan and irresponsible when I wrote that eating more fruit and vegetables and less refined, processed food could reduce the risk of some cancers. I was vilified for recommending garlic, oily fish, blueberries, prunes and cranberry juice as protection against heart disease. Yet now the wheel has come full circle and every cancer research body advises eating more fruit and vegetables and less meat. Research published as recently as December 2004 highlights the benefit of eating the right foods to prevent heart disease.

You don't need to wait for the scientists to catch up with common sense. There are no side effects from eating good food. This book proves that eating matters, food matters and above all, enjoyment matters. As much as we all have to eat to live, a little bit of living to eat matters, too.

shopping for good health

'You are what you eat' goes the proverb, and of course it's true. Unfortunately, what most people don't realize is that you're also what you *don't* eat. Despite a mountain of information about food, cooking, nutrition and health, messages get confused; in my surgery I see an ever-growing number of people who are either overfed but undernourished or are so busy trying to follow every piece of food advice they read or hear that they end up underfed as well as undernourished.

Yet how do you choose the right superfoods amid so many conflicting messages? Don't eat eggs – eat eggs; eat margarine – no, eat butter; eat soya – don't eat soya; you need salt – you don't; chocolate is good – chocolate is bad; eat meat – be vegetarian… It's easy to be confused and alarmed by each new report that makes the headlines. What you must ask when reading these stories is who's behind them; who stands to gain by changing public attitudes and eating habits? After all, in the first half of the twentieth century, mothers managed fairly well without an army of dieticians, nutritionists (qualified and bogus) and health experts. They relied on common sense, seasonal availability and the skills their own mothers passed on to raise healthy, well-fed families.

the three-bag system

It's easy to ensure you get a balanced diet if you use what I call the 'three-bag' trick when you go shopping. The size of the bags depends on how many people you're shopping for, but the proportions always stay the same. Fill one bag with the healthy starchy foods: wholemeal bread, brown rice, pasta, beans, wholegrain cereals like porridge, muesli, Shredded Wheat, Weetabix, whole-wheat flakes and of course, potatoes. The second bag should overflow with fruits, vegetables and salads. Frozen veg is fine if it's more convenient to your lifestyle, but make sure you include dried fruits, fresh nuts and seeds. The third bag is a bit more difficult. Just imagine that it has three separate bags inside: two the same size, which take up most of the space, and a third but much smaller bag. Fill the first with cheese, milk, yogurt and eggs, then the second with meat, fish, poultry or alternative vegetarian protein such as tofu, quorn or textured vegetable protein (TVP). The last tiny bag is reserved for treats like cream, biscuits, sweets, chocolates and sticky buns.

While you're shopping you should also give plenty of thought to the hidden additives found in any canned or processed foods. Read all labels to keep your salt intake as low as possible. Better yet, throw away the salt cellar and use more fresh herbs in your cooking; they not only taste good but have wonderful medicinal benefits. Sage, for example, improves the digestion of fats. Mint is a powerful antacid and prevents indigestion. Basil calms you down and makes you feel good. Bay leaves are good for chest infections. Garlic lowers cholesterol... the list goes on and on.

making the most of what you buy

Divide your dinner plate the same way and you'll have the healthiest possible diet. Following this scheme means you'll get at least half your calories from good carbohydrates, no more than a third of them from fat, and between ten and twelve percent from protein. By adding a couple of glasses of wine a day, your calories from alcohol will be less than ten percent and won't exceed the safe number of daily units. These proportions work for everyone unless there are specific medical reasons for eating differently. And this isn't hair-shirt time; you can still enjoy fresh cream on your strawberries, a piece of chocolate with your evening coffee or a delicious gooey dessert once in a while.

Sticking with that theme, let me state once and for all that bread, potatoes, rice, pasta and cereals are *not* fattening or unhealthy. It's what you do to them that makes the difference. Potatoes drizzled with olive oil, sprinkled with rosemary and roasted in the oven are wonderful. Pasta with tomato, vegetable or fish sauces is great food. Good wholemeal bread with a thin smear of butter is delicious and highly nutritious.

'A little of what you fancy does you good' is another of the truest proverbs. The occasional indulgence does no harm to your body – and a great deal of good for your soul. After all, eating should be about enjoyment, not guilt.

organic food: is it worth it?

As a student at the British College of Naturopathy and Osteopathy in the late 1950s and early '60s, I was introduced to the concept of organic eating. Being an osteopath and naturopath at that time was considered cranky enough, but to talk about 'organic' anything put me firmly in the lunatic fringe as far as the medical and scientific establishment was concerned.

So why do I insist on choosing the organic route? For three major reasons. Firstly because it's safe – a fact that should figure in the ultimate criteria for any superfood. No one in his or her right mind trusts government or industry assurances that agrochemical residues in food are 'safe'. We've all heard too many of these assurances and then seen the dire outcome with salmonella, listeria and BSE. The Ministry of Agriculture, Fisheries and Food has always been the friend of the farmer and the chemical industry, not the consumer – yet it's the consumer who carries the can when things go wrong. The official assumptions on safety do not hold water, especially when the precautionary principle of proving safety rather than demonstrating minimal risk, is not applied.

Secondly, I opt for organics because I have grave concerns for the survival of our planet. I was lucky enough to meet Rachel Carson, author of *Silent Spring*, the book that first raised awareness in the general public of the way in which agrochemicals were damaging biodiversity. As far back as the 1950s, she was aware that tiny doses of chemical residues worked their way through the food chain until the birds of prey were finally killed off. Biodiversity is the key to the earth's future, and therefore crucial to our own. In the UK, we've already seen an alarming decline of common birds, and our wild plants and flowers are following suit; Northamptonshire has lost ninety-three species of plants in the last sixty-five years and Gloucestershire, Middlesex, Cambridgeshire, Durham and Leicestershire are losing wild flora just as rapidly. Even rural Norfolk has lost thirty-three species in the last hundred years. And with the plants go the insects, bees and butterflies which depend on them and which are vital for pollination.

Thirdly, I am appalled by the prospect of GM foods. In spite of all the safety assurances given out on both sides of the Atlantic, there have already been disasters. At the end of 2000, for example, the American government forced the Kraft Foods corporation to recall millions of packets of taco pasta shells because the corn used in their manufacture was contaminated with a GM strain licensed only for animal feed. This modified variety doesn't break down by cooking and is not digested by gastric juices. It consequently poses a severe allergy threat and is also likely to be carcinogenic to humans.

In contrast, certified organic products are not only free of agrochemicals because they're grown that way, they're also free of artificial colourings, flavourings, additives, sweeteners and the thousands of other unwanted and unnecessary chemicals manufacturers add to food to enhance their profits.

the conscientious consumer

As consumers, we know we're making our voices heard when high-street supermarkets have been forced into ever-expanding ranges of organic goods, when whole chains of shops ban GM ingredients in their own-label products, and most of all when the agrochemical industry launches spurious attacks on organic food with laughable claims that it's dangerous because it may have bugs on it due to being fertilized with manure.

Yet we must remain vigilant in the way we shop – both for our health's sake and for that of the planet. Every time you purchase an organic product, you're not only ensuring that you get goo-quality, nutritious and unadulterated food, you're actually helping to reduce global warming by saving the energy used to produce harmful agrochemicals.

At the moment, we in the UK – unlike consumers in the US – still have a choice when it comes to buying non-GM food, but it is a choice we must continue to exercise if we want to keep it. For our own health and the health of the planet we live in, I'd say the cost is more than worth it.

taking the waters

While examining superfoods, it's all too easy to overlook the ultimate super beverage: water. Water is one of the most powerful and easily available of all natural medicines. Used by man in hot springs, cold springs, sulphur springs, as seawater, river water, mountain water, it has provided external as well as internal therapy. The whole art of hydrotherapy – using showers, baths of different temperatures, steam and alternate hot and cold bathing – has been part of the history of healing.

From the Turkish baths of the Ottoman Empire and the great bathhouses of the Roman Empire to the modern sophisticated spa, we've used water to bathe away our spiritual and emotional problems as well as to soothe our physical aches and pains. Yet most important of all is the water we *drink* – and few people drink enough. Kidney problems, cystitis, migraine, headaches, skin disorders, constipation... they may all have their roots in a lack of fluid intake. The huge rise in the popularity of mineral waters has helped make people more aware of water, which we so often take for granted.

Mineral waters not only taste good, they have health-giving properties as well. I've been a mineral-water fan ever since I was taught the medicinal value of them as a student of naturopathy. I'm delighted to see the phenomenal increase in their popularity. It doesn't surprise me, however, when you consider the life history of much of our tap water. Nearly all of it is recycled, and if you live in London, New York or any other big city, yours could be the seventh pair of kidneys that your glass of Adam's ale passes through! Also, many of the chemicals used in farming today seep into the ground to pollute and contaminate water: insecticides, pesticides, fungicides, herbicides, growth hormones and even antibiotics.

This wasn't always the case. In Victorian times, people flocked to Bath, Buxton, Leamington, Cheltenham and Harrogate in the UK, to Evian, Vichy, Baden Baden and Sangermini in Europe, to Hot Springs, Calistoga, Saratoga Springs and Poland Spring in the US to 'take the waters'. Now, more than a hundred years later, we are rediscovering their taste and value, yet what is the difference between them?

mineral waters

These must come from a single underground source and be free from dangerous bacteria and polluting chemicals. The waters can only be filtered and sterilized by ultraviolet light, and though some are naturally gassy, carbon dioxide may be added to still waters to make them fizzy. Labels must list the mineral content.

spring and table waters

These may come from a spring or out of a tap connected to your local water authority as long as they're safe to drink. The source doesn't have to be identified; in fact, it may be a mixture of different waters and the label doesn't have to declare the mineral content.

restaurant bottled waters

These may be nothing more than tap water which has been through a plumbed-in filtration system to remove the taste of chlorine and some minerals. Unless you like the taste of a particular bottled water, ask for a large jug of iced water and give it a good stir to remove chlorine.

Whether you choose a mineral water or water from the tap, what matters most to your health is how much you drink. Aim for a minimum of one litre a day, but if you really want a clear skin, bright eyes and happy kidneys, add another couple of glasses. And don't forget that any journey of more than around four hours is a risk for deep-vein thrombosis (DVT). Although flying gets all the publicity, it's just as bad in a car, coach or train if you don't get up and move around, wriggle your toes, tighten and relax your calf muscles, and drink extra water while you're travelling to reduce the possibility of blood clots.

A word of warning. Although bottled waters only contain minute quantities of minerals, anyone with high blood pressure or heart disease should still choose low-sodium waters as a safety precaution.

popular waters

highland spring (still)

Source	The Ochil Hills, Perthshire
Calcium content (mg/l)	39
Magnesium content (mg/l)	15
Sodium content (mg/l)	9
Total mineral content	Very low
Taste	Clean, fresh

Comments This is one of the best-selling of the British waters. It has a clean, fresh taste and is good to drink on its own, slightly chilled. Low in sodium and nitrates, this is suitable for those with heart and kidney problems. I like this one and often recommend it to patients.

buxton natural mineral water

Source	Buxton, Derbyshire
Calcium content (mg/l)	55
Magnesium content (mg/l)	19
Sodium content (mg/l)	24
Total mineral content	Low
Taste	Very light, clean

Comments Comes from an underground reservoir almost 5,000 feet deep. It comes out of the ground at a temperature of 27.8°C (82°F) and was drunk by medieval pilgrims and Mary Queen of Scots. My favourite of all the British waters, it's still available at St Ann's Well, the public drinking fountain at Buxton.

san pellegrino

Source	Italian Alps
Calcium content (mg/l)	203
Magnesium content (mg/l)	56.9
Sodium content (mg/l)	46.5
Total mineral content	Medium
Taste	A refreshing, distinctive flavour

Comments Leonardo da Vinci drank this water which is still, very warm and boasting a metallic aftertaste as it came straight from the spring. Modern carbonated water loses most of the mineral flavour which is replaced by a sparkling crispness.

spa (still)

Source	Spa Reine, Belgium
Calcium content (mg/l)	3.5
Magnesium content (mg/l)	1.3
Sodium content (mg/l)	3
Total mineral content	Very low
Taste	Just a hint of flavour

Comments This Belgian variety has been exported for more than 400 years. It has a very low salt content and is one of the best-known mineral waters in the world. Peter the Great, Charles II and Disraeli were all fans. Spa is perfect for those on a low-salt diet.

volvic

Source	The Clairvic Spring, France
Calcium content (mg/l)	9.9
Magnesium content (mg/l)	6.1
Sodium content (mg/l)	9.4
Total mineral content	Low
Taste	Very plain hardly flavoured pure water

Comments This mountain water, from the deserted volcanic region of the Auvergne, takes many years to drain through the basalt rocks. It's best drunk chilled. Thanks to its low sodium and calcium and reasonable magnesium content, it's good for making up baby foods and for skin problems. Some say that Volvic makes the best coffee.

evian

Source	Evian, Lake Geneva
Calcium content (mg/l)	78
Magnesium content (mg/l)	24
Sodium content (mg/l)	5
Total mineral content	Low
Taste	Pure, very clean taste

Comments Ideal for the whole family, and the only water the French government recommends for mixing baby foods. The spa at Evian has been famous since the eighteenth century as *the* place for the treatment of kidney stones and urinary infections. Evian water takes fifteen years to filter down from the Alpine snows to the spring in the town. More than 200 laboratory checks are made each day at the bottling plant, and thousands of French men and women visit the Lakeside Spa each year, to take the cure and drink the water – all paid for by the state health service! This is the biggest seller of all still waters in its native France.

badoît (naturally sparkling)

Source	Badoît, Saint-Galmier, France
Calcium content (mg/l)	200
Magnesium content (mg/l)	100
Sodium content (mg/l)	160
Total mineral content	medium
Taste	slightly alkaline and very refreshing

Comments This wonderful water was the first ever bottled in France. It emerges from a 500m fissure in the granite, slightly sparkling, with its high bicarbonate content making it the best of all sparkling waters to drink with food. It contains 1mg per litre of fluoride, enough to give the local children better teeth than in any of the surrounding villages. The Romans built a bathhouse here and local doctors endorsed the benefits of the water in the seventeenth century. When Louis Pasteur was working in Italy in the late 1800s, he used to order fifty bottles at a time.

vichy (naturally fizzy)

Source:Vichy, France	
Calcium content (mg/l)	100
Magnesium content (mg/l)	9
Sodium content (mg/l)	1,200
Total mineral content	High
Taste	Very alkaline, very slightly fizzy

Comments The most fashionable and elegant of all the spas in the 1800s. Vichy is the water for digestive problems, rheumatism and kidney stones. Frequented by Napoléon the third, and most of the crowned heads of Europe, Vichy is once again a fashionable place. The elegant old hotels have been restored, the original thermal treatment centre updated and aimed at the new health-conscious market. If you can't get to Vichy, at least try the water.

superfoods

From almonds to yogurt, each of the following 100 superfoods possesses its own particular health benefit. Everyone knows how healthy broccoli, cabbage and spinach are, but you'll be delighted to learn that every woman should enjoy a glass of beer, that avocados are a superfood for your skin, and that potatoes are low in calories, bursting with nutrients – and they aren't fattening at all. For a real surprise, read on to discover what makes prunes the most protective of all foods.

almonds

Almonds are not only delicious, they're symbolic, too. In many cultures, almonds in some form – shelled, roasted, or sugared – are traditional fare at festive occasions such as weddings and confirmations. Of course, the healthiest way to eat them is freshly shelled and natural, but because of their high nutritional value they're ideal finely ground and added to soups, desserts or porridge for anyone who is convalescing or having problems with eating.

The two varieties are sweet and bitter almonds, but the most commonly eaten are the sweet ones. Bitter almonds contain toxic prussic acid and should never be eaten raw, as this poison is only destroyed by heating. Bitter almonds are used mainly to make almond oil. They're rich in protein, heart-protective mono-unsaturated fats and vital minerals like zinc, magnesium, potassium and iron, as well as some B vitamins. Since they're also high in oxalic and phytic acid, which combine with these minerals to carry them out of your body, you should eat them at the same time as vitamin C-rich foods for maximum absorption.

Of all the nuts, almonds contain the most calcium and twenty percent protein; weight for weight, that's a third more protein than eggs. Almond oil is wonderfully soothing to the skin as it's rich in vitamin E and ideal for preventing stretch marks and healing scars.

Almond milk is a classic sickroom drink, used by herbalists for the relief of chest infections and digestive problems. Soak 50g of whole almonds in tepid water then skin them and pound them (you can use a food processor) with some of a litre of water. Add the paste to the rest of the water, stir in a tablespoonful of honey, strain through muslin.

Almond butter makes a highly nutritious alternative to peanut butter and is easy to make at home. An electric coffee grinder is ideal; fill it with a handful of nuts, grind a bit adding a little almond oil, and continue until you have the desired texture. It will keep for up to three days in the fridge.

angelica

Although angelica is known mostly in its crystallized form as a decoration for cakes, it has a long history of medicinal use. Chinese angelica is a household remedy for women, relieving menstrual discomfort, reducing pain and encouraging the regularity of the cycle. American angelica, sometimes called 'bellyache root', is effective for wind and heartburn, and European angelica is traditionally used for liver disorders and arthritis; it's also a gentle stimulant.

Although used for centuries in China, angelica was not a recognized medicine in Europe until the fifteenth century, when tea made from the leaves was used for bronchitis, catarrh, loss of appetite and as a gentle stimulant. Its pungent flavour is used in some liqueurs such as Benedictine, and its iron content makes the bitter leaves a valuable and interesting addition to cooking.

Sprinkle a few angelica leaves into your bath, to stimulate and relieve aching joints. Hang a bag of crushed leaves in your car as a brilliant air freshener; it will also help keep you awake.

anise

Anise was introduced to Britain in the fourteenth century and taken to the US by the pilgrims, where it became an important crop of medicinal value for the Shakers. Also known as aniseed, it's from the same family as cumin, dill and fennel, and its flavour and medicinal value come from the essential oils anethole and estragole. The seeds relieve hard, dry coughs and thin congested mucus; they also improve breathing.

To make aniseed tea, crush a teaspoon of seeds and add them to a cup of boiling water. The digestive benefits of anise are legendary, which is why it is often used in the preparation of liqueurs and aperitifs. It can also stimulate lactation in nursing mothers.

Use anise as a delicious flavouring for sweet as well as savoury dishes such as cakes, biscuits, soups, stews and casseroles.

apples

According to an ancient proverb, 'If you can plant only one tree in your garden, this should be an apple tree.' How true. An apple a day may keep the doctor away, but two is a real tonic for your heart and circulation. Apples are rich in a soluble fibre known as pectin, which helps eliminate cholesterol and protects against environmental pollutants. Two apples a day can lower your cholesterol by ten percent, and the pectin also combines with toxic heavy metals and removes them from the body.

Apples also contain malic and tartaric acids, which improve digestion and the breakdown of fats, so the traditional apple sauce with pork, or sage and apple stuffing in goose, or an apple with cheese not only tastes good but does you good in other ways.

You wouldn't normally think of apples as aromatherapy, but somewhat surprisingly, even their natural perfume can lower your blood pressure and calm the nerves. Medically, they're helpful in the relief of the pain of gout, rheumatism and arthritis, and because of their cleansing properties, they will help you feel better the morning after a night on the town.

Naturopaths have always valued apples as a treatment for diarrhoea and food poisoning. Grated apples, mixed with honey and left in a bowl until they turn brown, make an excellent remedy for diarrhoea. For food poisoning, they're a vital ingredient of the BRAT diet: a traditional method of dealing with food poisoning. It consists of bananas, boiled rice, apples, dry toast, plenty of water and nothing else until the symptoms subside.

The vitamin C found in apples is an immune- booster, and research shows that apple juice can kill a wide range of viruses. As the sugar in this fruit is mostly fructose, it's broken down slowly by the body and helps maintain blood sugar at a steady level, thus avoiding hypoglycaemia and sugar cravings.

apricots

The health benefits of apricots were first recognized by an ancient tribe called the Hunzas. They lived high in the Himalayas where apricots, both fresh and dried, were a major part of their staple diet. It is known that they had exceptionally long lives; many lived beyond 100.

We now know that apricots are a rich source of betacarotenes, which the body converts into vitamin A – essential for immunity, skin, vision and healthy mucous membranes. Fresh and dried apricots should form a regular part of the diet for anyone with infections, skin problems, with, or at risk of, cancer (e.g. smokers). Because they also contain a wide range of protective plant chemicals, they're important in the prevention of many different types of cancer, especially of the mouth.

Due to their high fibre content, apricots are one of the best foods for the treatment and prevention of constipation. Another major ingredient is potassium, which is heart-protective, helps reduce blood pressure, encourages the elimination of salt, and consequently will reduce fluid retention. They're also a rich source of well-absorbed iron, so they're of triple benefit during pregnancy thanks to the iron, the reduction of fluid retention and the prevention of constipation, all of which can present problems.

Dried apricots make a brilliant snack; they're filling, nourishing and a source of instant as well as slow-release energy. They're a perfect addition to shakes and smoothies, and fresh apricots make delicious, health-giving juice. If you're lucky enough to find really ripe, succulent fruits, remove the stones, put them in a blender and purée. Add some ice-cubes, some sparkling mineral water and you have a refreshing drink. To spoil yourself, add Champagne – much more interesting than Buck's Fizz.

Dried apricots should be bright orange; the darker they are, the less betacarotene they have. Most dried apricots are preserved with sulphur dioxide, which can trigger asthma attacks, so rinse well with warm water before eating.

artichokes

There are two types of artichoke, totally unrelated, but both with medicinal benefits. Globe artichokes belong to the thistle family and they grow throughout the Mediterranean. Jerusalem artichokes come from North America but reached France during the seventeenth century; they are related to sunflowers.

Both artichokes contain little starch, but instead they're rich in a substance known as inulin. The body deals with this in the same way as it copes with fibre, as it isn't broken down during normal digestion but ends up in the large bowel where colonies of probiotic bacteria ferment the inulin. This chemical has all the benefits of fibre but, unfortunately, it can be the cause of excessive wind.

If you're lucky enough to be invited to eat in a French home and the main course is something fairly rich and fatty, you will almost certainly be served globe artichoke as the first course. This wonderful vegetable is a huge source of cynarine, a bitter-tasting substance that increases the flow of bile and improves liver function. The result is better digestion and breakdown of all types of fat, because the extra bile emulsifies the fat into tiny globules – just like washing up liquid on your greasy dishes – which increases the surface area exposed to digestive juices and speeds up the whole process.

Herbalists have long used extracts of globe artichoke (as well as its close relative, the milk thistle) in the treatment of all sorts of liver and gall-bladder disorders. But it's also valuable as a diuretic and can help lower cholesterol levels. If you're daft enough to end up with a hangover, extracts containing cynarine (or, if you can face it, a whole artichoke) will make you feel better than you deserve.

Jerusalem artichokes are small, potato-like tubers that make wonderful soup and are delicious hot or cold as a vegetable. Both varieties are the easiest thing in the world to grow and produce abundant crops, so if you've got the space, plant some.

asparagus

This is one of the world's great food treats, with a reputation of being a gourmet delicacy. In restaurants, it's always expensive, and its health benefits are diminished by the addition of rich sauces, piles of Parmesan cheese or far too much melted butter – all of which are sources of artery-clogging saturated fat.

If there's any space in your garden for an asparagus bed, have one. Although the first couple of years take time and effort, the reward of fresh spears, homemade soup, or real asparagus omelettes for the next ten years requires very little work.

Asparagus has been used for medicinal purposes for the last 500 years, but it has been cultivated as a vegetable for more than two millennia. Although it's helpful in the relief of urinary infections, constipation, arthritis and rheumatism, its most powerful effect is as a diuretic. A natural chemical called asparagine is responsible for this action, as you'll soon realize within half an hour of eating a portion. Not only will your output of urine increase, but it will have a distinctive smell that is unmistakable (but perfectly normal).

Over a thousand years ago, Dioscorides, the pioneering Greek doctor, used asparagus to treat both liver and kidney disorders, but it took 1,500 years before it was widely used as a medicine again. Although it is a great help in the relief of arthritis and rheumatism, avoid asparagus like the plague if you suffer from gout. It contains a group of chemicals called purines which can trigger episodes and greatly aggravate the pain if you're already having an attack.

Don't waste anything when you prepare and cook asparagus, as the bottom ends which you cut off can go into homemade stock or soups, and the cooking water can be drunk or added to soups and gravies for its diuretic properties. It's also ideal for women who suffer with swollen ankles, fingers and breasts with every period.

avocados

Almost every single woman I know believes that avocados are fattening. In fact, they're a fabulous food containing a little protein, some starch, heart-protective mono-unsaturated fat, plenty of potassium, and vitamins A, B, C and E.

They've been grown in South America for 8,000 years, where indigenous tribes used the fruit, dried leaves, fresh leaves, rind, bark and the seed medicinally. Calorie for calorie, avocados offer super nutrition, and the high content of oleic acid they contain makes them a powerful antioxidant. Consequently, they protect us against heart disease, strokes and some forms of cancer.

Puréed avocado is an ideal food for anyone who is unwell or recovering from illness or surgery; it is especially valuable for ill children. It's easy to digest, and a rich source of natural antibiotic and antifungal chemicals. You may think that guacamole is just an excuse for eating lots of tacos, but in fact, it is a dish that provides loads of energy, important amounts of protein, and an extremely valuable source of naturally protective chemicals.

Because they're rich in vitamin E, avocados are important in the diet of anyone planning conception or with fertility problems. Their B vitamin content will help you cope with stress, tension and anxiety. Because they contain vitamin B_6 they're ideal for women suffering from PMS, and should be eaten regularly in the ten days leading up to the next period.

Another totally different benefit is the way in which avocados help improve and maintain healthy skin. The natural oils and vitamins A and E are antioxidant, and thus prevent premature ageing of the skin and the formation of wrinkles. When applied externally, a purée of avocado mixed with live yogurt makes a fabulous face mask for cleansing and nourishing. It will increase the amount of collagen, which helps to reduce existing wrinkles and maintains clear and youthful-looking skin.

bananas

These are nature's superb fast food, packed with nutrients: potassium, zinc, iron, folic acid and calcium. They're also a good source of pectin, a soluble fibre that improves the elimination of toxins. Sadly, a very common perception is that they're fattening, but this is far from the truth; the average banana supplies fewer than 100 calories.

Because of their combination of instant and slow-release energy as well as cramp-preventing potassium, bananas are the perfect snack for anyone engaged in strenuous exercise. They're also highly protective against high blood pressure, heart disease and fluid retention. Bananas are the perfect replacement for high-sugar and high-fat nibbles when your energy starts to wane during a busy day at work or leisure, and the vitamin B_6 they contain means they're extremely useful for alleviating the symptoms of PMS.

The starch in bananas is not easily digested, which is why they should only be eaten ripe, when most of the starch has turned to sugar. This happens when the skin becomes speckled brown. Big brother to the banana is the plantain, which should only be eaten cooked, as they're virtually indigestible raw.

As long ago as the 1930s, research showed that bananas were both preventive and curative for stomach ulcers, a fact widely touted in ancient Indian folklore. Traditional practitioners, however, found that the best treatment for ulcers is flour made from dried green plantains and made into a very thin porridge. This fact has now been confirmed by modern scientific investigation.

Throughout India, Africa and South America, plantains are used much like potatoes. They're a major source of energy and are wonderful to eat boiled, fried or baked, and go particularly well with fish.

Because the fibre found in ripe bananas and cooked plantains is so easily digestible, they help in the treatment of both constipation and diarrhoea. A little-known fact: sticking a piece of banana skin, yellow side out, over a wart or verruca will speed its demise.

barley

Sadly, barley is a much-neglected grain which has amazing nutritional and health properties. The grains contain natural soothing lubricants that have a direct healing action on mucous membranes, which explains its traditional use for the treatment of sore throats, oesophagitis, gastritis and colitis. Barley contains calcium, potassium, and plenty of B-complex vitamins, so it's good if you're feeling stressed, exhausted or recovering from illness.

Lemon barley water is a traditional remedy for cystitis and other urinary problems. Add a tablespoon of washed pot barley to half a litre of water and two quartered unwaxed lemons. Bring to the boil, cover, and simmer for thirty minutes. Strain, refrigerate and drink several glasses a day.

The Latin name for barley is *Hordeum*, and to Romans it was such a strengthening food that gladiators ate it regularly – which is why they were called *Hordearii*, or 'barley-eaters'. The great fourth-century Roman gastronome, Apicius, lists several recipes for barley soups, including *Tisanam* and *Tisanam sic facies,* which were formulated to the Roman medical idea of *tisanam*: barley waters used as medicine, which is where the modern word 'tisane' originated.

Barley is the oldest cultivated cereal. You can benefit from this highly strengthening and protective grain by using barley flour in biscuits, bread and cakes, adding barley flakes to breakfast cereals, and using plenty of the whole grains in soups, stews and casseroles. Barley is rich in soluble fibre and other natural chemicals that reduce cholesterol levels and specifically protect against many forms of cancer. Modern research has shown that barley inhibits the manufacture of cholesterol in the liver as well as increasing its elimination from the body.

Pot barley is highly superior to the more widely available pearl barley, as it retains much more of the fibres and gut-soothing chemicals. Although more processed forms do provide good quantities of minerals, they contain considerably smaller amounts of vitamins.

basil

The traditional ingredient of Mediterranean tomato dishes and an important component of pesto sauce, basil is one of the most versatile and useful culinary herbs. Although everyone thinks of this as a Mediterranean plant, it actually started life in the east, where it is native to India, other parts of south Asia and areas of the Middle East. Basil came to Europe early on, and is mentioned by the classical writers of the first two centuries. In fact, the name 'basil' is derived from the Greek *basilikon phuton*, which means 'a kingly herb'.

A variety called holy basil is considered sacred by the Hindus, and in Christianity it is believed to have appeared growing around Christ's tomb after the Resurrection. You'll often find it growing wild around remote churches in Greece, where it's sometimes used to prepare holy water.

The leaves contain volatile oils, especially linalool, limonene and estragole, which account for the medicinal properties of this herb. It relieves flatulence, is an aid to digestion, and its antiseptic properties are said to benefit acne.

If you want a good night's sleep, there's nothing better than the delicate flavour of basil. It's a mild sedative and acts as the perfect evening snack for insomniacs. Simply tear up three or four leaves into small pieces, and add to a sandwich of lettuce and tomato.

There are a number of different varieties, all with slightly different flavours: peppermint, lemon, cinnamon, purple and bush basil. It's really worth growing your own because the flavour of dried basil doesn't even come close to the real thing freshly picked from your window box, garden or greenhouse.

In the Provence region of France, pesto is known as *pistou*, and there is nothing more calming or relaxing at the end of a really stressful day than a bowl of traditional *soupe ou pistou*. Any decent French cookery book will give you the recipe. If you're having a barbecue, try rubbing exposed skin with a basil leaf – it's a great insect repellent.

bay leaves

Laurus nobilis is the Latin name for the bay tree. Dedicated to Apollo and used in crowns awarded to emperors, scholars and athletes, this is a prized herb.

Traditional in French *bouquet garni*, the leaves have antiseptic properties, improve digestion and impart flavour. They're a wonderful addition to most soups, stews and casseroles, and indispensable in marinades. They're also great as flavour enhancers in milk-based puddings – but make sure you remove them before eating.

The leaves contain the volatile oils geraniol, cineole and eugenol, and when used in recipes they stimulate digestive juices and improve nutrient absorption from food. This is a particularly good herb for anyone recovering from serious illness as it helps optimize nutrition.

Do try growing one of these evergreens in a sheltered spot in your garden, as the fresh leaves contain more of the essential oils and have a much more subtle flavour.

bean sprouts

Bean sprouts supply abundant vitamins and minerals. They're cheap, easy to grow and guaranteed free of chemicals if you do it yourself. I always think of sprouted beans (and seeds, too, for that matter) as 'future foods'. Inside the bean are all the nutrients needed to trigger the growth of the next generation of plants. Sprouting increases the amount of available vitamins. Vitamin B_2 in oats was increased by 2,000 percent by the time green leaves appeared, B_6 was up 500 percent, and folic acid 600 percent. Sprouted wheat contained 600 percent more vitamin C than wheat grain.

Aduki, mung and soya beans, chickpeas, barley and wheat are all easy to grow at home. Soak in warm water for twelve hours. Drain, put in a jam jar, and cover with muslin. Keep the jar in a warm, dark place. Rinse twice a day and enjoy your delicious, nutrient-packed harvest. If you want to be posh, you can buy special sprouting kits.

beans

Dried beans or pulses are part of the legume family and the second-largest group of foods forming man's diet. They're low in fat and salt, cholesterol-free, and a rich source of proteins, starches, vitamins, minerals and fibre. They're also cheap and can be stored for long periods. Pound for pound, they contain almost as much protein as fillet steak – at a fraction of the cost and with many more health benefits. Beans help reduce cholesterol in the blood and are rich in essential minerals, B vitamins and folic acid. They protect against heart disease, circulatory problems and bowel cancer, and they're a valuable source of slow-release energy, making them an excellent food for diabetics. Beans also contain plant hormones called phytoestrogens, which protect against breast and prostate cancers and dramatically reduce the risk of osteoporosis as long as they are part of your regular staple diet.

Dried beans are the cheapest, but many need soaking before cooking, so canned beans are a great alternative; rinse well to remove the salt. Soya beans are the best vegetable source of protein and can also be made into tofu, soya milk, soya cheese and soya flour. But they also have the highest content of phytoestrogens, and the strongest antioxidant activity, which protects against heart disease and cancer.

All beans are valuable. Some of their individual properties include:

Aduki	Fibre, magnesium, potassium, zinc
Baked beans	Fibre, iron, selenium, iodine (but beware the salt)
Black-eyed	Fibre, selenium, folate
Butter	Fibre, potassium, iron
Chickpeas	Fibre, calcium, iron, zinc
Haricot	Fibre, iron
Kidney	Fibre, potassium, zinc
Mung	Less starch, more folate
Pinto	Potassium, fibre, folate

Worried about the 'flatulence factor'? Add some summer savory for its anti-wind effect.

beef

In early English history, beef was reserved for the ruling Normans; the poor Anglo-Saxons went without until after the thirteenth century. The traditional roast beef of old England, a genuine Aberdeen Angus sirloin or a homemade steak-and-kidney pie taste wonderful and provide essential nutrients, including protein, iron, B vitamins and minerals.

Sadly, these dishes can also be nutritional disasters. We eat too much meat, and reducing consumption of red meat also reduces the risks of bowel cancer, high blood pressure and heart disease. So if you like beef, eat less but buy the best. That means organic. The fat of cattle that have been free-ranged on organic pastures contains conjugated linoleic acid, or CLA, a substance that is almost completely absent in intensively reared animals. Not only does this natural fat have powerful cancer-fighting properties, it also stimulates the conversion of our stored fat into energy, thus helping to control weight.

Non-organic beef will contain chemical residues from its feed and, although they are now banned in most of Europe, it is still likely to contain illegal hormones and antibiotics. Beef imported from other parts of the world will almost certainly contain chemicals you don't want in your body.

Cooking is the key to healthy beef-eating. Always roast joints on a trivet so that the fat drips through into the pan; it's the worst sort of saturated fat that clogs your arteries. Grill or griddle steaks for the same reason, and when making stews or casseroles, remove most of the surface fat before cooking.

If you like burgers, you should make your own, but even then they must be cooked right through to avoid food poisoning. The good news is you can still enjoy rare steaks and roast beef as long as the outside of the meat has been thoroughly cooked. That's where the bugs are until you mince the beef, when they end up on the inside.

beer

If you find the idea of 'laddettes' swigging pints of bitter unappealing, think again. There are plenty of reasons for women to indulge in this most traditional of all British drinks.

Beer is one of the best nutritional sources of the mineral silicon, which is essential for building strong bones and for the prevention of osteoporosis. Even more importantly, it's easier for the body to use the silicon in beer than in almost any other foodstuff. As little as half a pint a day could help prevent the dangerous osteoporosis that causes more than 200,000 fractures every year – most of them in women.

There's even more good news, particularly for women, as the latest evidence from Japan reveals that the hops used in traditional brewing are a good source of phytoestrogens: the natural plant hormones that protect against osteoporosis. If you really want to strengthen your bones, next time you go to a pub, have a ploughman's lunch and a glass of beer. The calcium in the cheese and natural ingredients in the beer make this the perfect bone-building meal.

This wonderful drink is also an excellent source of B vitamins, notably B_{12}, B_6 and folic acid, which many women lack in their diets. As a bonus, hops have a natural antibiotic action that kills the *Helicobacter pylori* bug, a common cause of stomach ulcers. For this reason, regular but modest beer-drinkers are much less likely to suffer from this problem.

Beer contains lots of potassium but very little sodium, so it's good for your blood pressure. Its high levels of magnesium and small quantities of calcium help to prevent kidney and gallstones, and a pint provides up to thirty percent of your daily fibre needs, thanks to the barley content. It's this special form of soluble fibre that prevents constipation and keeps your cholesterol low.

Beer is nature's tonic. It looks good, tastes good and really does you good.

beetroot

Ancient Greeks revered beetroot as a medicine and offered it as a tribute to Apollo in the temple at Delphi. Although there's not yet a great deal of scientific evidence to support the medicinal value of the beetroot, there is more than enough folklore and herbalists' knowledge to recommend it. Eat beetroot at least once a week for specific therapeutic benefits.

In Romany medicine, beetroot juice was used as a blood-builder, and in Russia and Eastern Europe, it is still used to increase resistance and to strengthen convalescents. Fresh, raw beet juice is a powerful blood-cleanser and tonic, and was valued for centuries as a digestive aid and liver stimulant.

In the traditional medicine of central Europe, beetroot has long been used in the treatment of cancer, and now modern research is beginning to explain its healing action. Some specific anti-carcinogens are bound to the red colouring matter, and it also increases the cellular uptake of oxygen by as much as 400 percent.

Beet greens are equally valuable, containing betacarotene and other carotenoids, lots of folate, potassium, some iron and vitamin C, all of which makes the roots and greens excellent for women planning pregnancy, women in general and anyone suffering from chronic fatigue syndromes.

A mixture of beetroot, carrot, apple and celery juice makes an excellent treatment for ME, Tired all the Time syndrome, chronic fatigue, glandular fever and other debilitating illnesses. Try taking a small wineglass of this delicious drink before each meal.

Beetroot is best eaten raw in a salad, boiled as a vegetable, baked in the oven or as traditional beetroot soup (borscht). Don't forget the leaves, which can be cooked like spinach.

And don't panic when you go to the loo. I've frequently been called at three in the morning by a patient whom I've put on the beetroot juice therapy to say they're passing blood in their urine or stool. It's only the beetroot's colouring.

blackberries

Although cultivated varieties are now available, nothing compares with the taste of freshly picked wild blackberries. They grow rampantly almost anywhere, and thanks to divine intervention, they're at their best at the same time as Bramley apples. The late summer/early autumn treat of apple and blackberry pie comes at just the right time to boost the immune system for the cold, wet days to come.

The ancient Greeks used blackberries to treat gout, and they're a good source of fibre. They're rich in vitamins E and C, so they're useful in the prevention and treatment of heart and circulatory problems and protective against cancers, degenerative diseases and infections.

Their astringent leaves contain antiseptic tannins, so chopped and used as tea they're an excellent mouthwash for gum problems and infections such as gingivitis, as well as an effective gargle for sore throats. An ounce of dried leaves in a pint of boiling water is an excellent remedy for diarrhoea; two cups a day is usually sufficient. A poultice of leaves macerated in boiling water and left to cool is a traditional remedy for scalds; the tannins act as an antiseptic and prevent secondary infection.

Try treating yourself to blackberry cordial with nutmeg, cloves and a little brandy for a real boost when you're feeling down. They're also an extremely good way of lowering high temperatures; simply soak fresh berries in apple cider vinegar for three days, strain through a sieve, add a pound of sugar for each pint of liquid, boil for five minutes and bottle when cool. One teaspoon of this mixture in a glass of water helps reduce fever and quench the thirst in adults and children.

Gathering blackberries used to be a great family outing that marked the end of summer but, sadly, few people seem to bother these days. The wild blackberry is food for free and collecting them is great exercise – but don't pick them from roadside hedges where they're likely to be contaminated by traffic fumes.

blackcurrants

The blackcurrant gets its proper name, *Ribes*, from an ancient Arabic word and has been used as both food and medicine for many centuries. These tart, uniquely flavoured berries are an exceptionally rich source of vitamin C, containing four times as much as an equivalent weight of oranges; 25g (1oz) will give you 60mg of this vital vitamin. The vitamin C in blackcurrants is particularly stable. French studies have shown that other substances in the fruit inhibit its oxidation and a syrup of blackcurrants loses only fifteen percent of its vitamin C in a year.

It's vitamin C that most people think of as the real medicinal value of this tiny berry, and it is a powerful antioxidant, protecting against heart disease, circulatory problems and all manner of infections. But blackcurrants also contain substantial amounts of potassium and very little sodium, so they help with water retention and are useful in the treatment of high blood pressure.

Pigments called anthocyanosides in their purple-black skins are antibacterial and have an anti-inflammatory action, which is why slowly sipped blackcurrant juice is an effective folk remedy for sore throats. To make it at home, simmer half a cup of blackcurrants in two cups of hot water for ten minutes, then strain and add some honey. Alternatively, add boiling water to a teaspoon of blackcurrant jelly. This powerful antibacterial effect is valuable in the treatment and prevention of food poisoning, as many of the bugs that trigger stomach upsets are destroyed by the anthocyanosides.

Blackcurrant leaves have important medical uses, too, as they contain volatile oils, tannins and more vitamin C. Put two teaspoons of chopped leaves in a glass of boiling water, cover and leave for ten minutes. Strain and use as a gargle for sore throats or as a mouthwash for painful ulcers. Two cups a day help relieve stress and anxiety as they affect the adrenal glands, stimulating the sympathetic nervous system.

blueberries

Blueberries grow as a small shrub with greenish berries that turn a rich purple as they ripen. Distinguishing between various members of this family is not always easy, but cranberries are very close relatives. Other members include bilberries, whortleberries, huckleberries and whinberries.

Blueberries are one of the most powerful health-protective foods. They help protect every cell in the body by their ability to neutralize damaging free-radical chemicals that are by-products of our own chemical processes and also the result of pollution. Thankfully, blueberries are now easily available. They should form a regular part of everyone's diet. Please don't just get them in muffins but sprinkle them fresh on your breakfast cereal, add them to fruit salads, turn them into smoothies along with low-fat yogurt, other berries and a banana. It's hard to believe anything tasting this good is also healthy, but it's a fact that blueberries help slow the ageing processes and protect against heart and circulatory disease and many forms of cancer.

Nutritionally speaking, blueberries are not very exciting, though they do contain reasonable amounts of vitamin C and small amounts of vitamin B_1, betacarotene and potassium. They're also a source of antibacterial anthocyanosides which have a tonic effect on blood vessels, making them good for varicose veins. Like cranberries, they also contain vegetable mucilage, which lines the urinary tract and prevents bacteria attaching themselves to the bladder wall. These antibacterial benefits help in the treatment of cystitis and other urinary infections.

In dried berries, the concentration of tannins and the other antibacterials is substantially increased. In Scandinavia, a traditional soup is made from dried blueberries and used as a simple but effective treatment for diarrhoea.

A traditional American folk remedy is made by soaking blueberries in brandy for three weeks, then straining off the berries. A teaspoonful several times a day is recommended for the treatment of food poisoning.

brazil nuts

Why do we only eat Brazil nuts at Christmas? My guess is that even most of these get thrown away unshelled. What a tragedy! These hugely nutritious nuts grow high in the crowns of some of the tallest Amazonian rainforest trees. Brazils have always been important in the diets of the indigenous tribes of the rain forest, and to this day they're collected from wild trees that grow in the forest, not specially grown plantations.

Strictly speaking, they are really seeds, not nuts, as they grow in large, round fruits a bit bigger than a cricket ball. Each fruit contains up to twenty-five nuts arranged like the segments of an orange, which is why they have their unique triangular shape. The fruit drops from the trees about fourteen months after flowering, and if nature is left to its own devices, it's gnawed open by the agouti, a large rodent who carries off the nuts and buries them in the ground.

Commercial harvesters collect the nuts early in the mornings between January and March, and hopefully get to them before the agoutis do. Each fruit can weigh up to 2.5kg and drops from around 200 feet with lethal force, but they're less likely to drop until later in the day.

Brazil nuts are high in fat – mostly the healthy poly- and mono-unsaturated varieties – and soon go rancid, so buy small quantities at a time. They're one of the richest of all sources of the essential mineral selenium, which is so deficient in the British diet. This vital mineral protects men against prostate cancer and women against breast cancer. It's also a vital nutrient to ensure a healthy heart. Unfortunately, the average amount in our daily diet is now only thirty micrograms and the minimum we need is seventy. Three or four each day will give you all you need.

Brazils are also a source of vitamins A, B_1, B_2 and niacin, and surprisingly, they also contain iodine, essential for the thyroid, with 100g supplying ten percent of your daily needs.

bread

Good bread really is 'the Staff of Life', but most people still believe that it's fattening. This is far from the truth, as it's a vital part of a healthy, balanced diet, and can help weight loss. 'How?' I hear you shouting. 'We've always been told to cut down on starch to lose weight.'

It's the *type* of starch that matters. If you stick to complex wholegrain starches like wholemeal bread, brown rice, pasta, oats and barley, they provide slow-release energy which prevents sugar cravings, plus they're extremely filling, which reduces hunger. They'll also give you protein, B vitamins, vitamin E, minerals and fibre.

If every shopper switched to wholemeal bread today, the health of the nation would start improving tomorrow. If you can't get the kids to eat it, make them sandwiches with one slice of decent white bread on top and wholemeal on the bottom; it usually works.

Six million loaves of processed, sliced, wrapped white bread are produced daily in the UK. Adverts tell us this tasteless, plastic-wrapped cotton wool is just as good as wholemeal. But is it? Wholemeal contains five times as much fibre, and valuable amounts of vitamin E, potassium, iron, zinc, copper, magnesium, thiamine, riboflavin, pantathenic acid, folic acid, pyridoxine and biotin. You'll also get ten times as much manganese, twice as much chromium and one-and-a-half times as much selenium.

Watch out for salt in commercial bread, as most manufacturers label it as 'grams of sodium per 100g'. Multiply this figure by 2.5, and you'll find out how much you're really getting – 530mg of sodium per 100g actually means 1.3g of salt from three slices. Your daily total shouldn't exceed 5g.

The best answer is to make your own, one of the most satisfying things you can ever do in a kitchen. But if you don't fancy all that kneading and pummelling (although it's a great way to get rid of anger and frustration), why not buy a bread machine? Either way, you control exactly what goes into your daily bread.

broccoli

Broccoli is a very rich source of carotenoids, especially betacarotene, which the body converts into vitamin A. Betacarotene and many of the other carotenoids are known to restrict the development and growth of cancer cells, and they play a vital role in the prevention of many types of cancer.

Ever since the scare over US President Reagan's bowel cancer, broccoli has become a four-star vegetable. The American National Cancer Institute advised a special diet for the president which included copious amounts of broccoli. Like other members of the cruciferous family of vegetables, it has been shown to have protective powers against cancer. (Other crucifers include cauliflower, kale, radishes, horseradish, cabbage, spring greens, turnips and Brussels sprouts). According to an analysis conducted by the US National Cancer Institute in 1987, six out of seven major population studies showed that the more cruciferous vegetables you eat, the lower your chances of developing cancer of the colon. Other cancers appeared to slow down as well.

A number of chemical compounds in the cruciferous vegetables have been identified as being responsible for this effect. Glucobrassicin and sinigrin are the major glucosinolates that are present in crucifers, and in response to cell damage they are converted to indoles. In Japan, where the incidence of colon cancer is extremely low, the average intake of glucosinolates is 100mg a day. In Britain, where there is a high incidence of colon cancer, the intake is less than a quarter of this amount.

Because of its potential to increase vitamin A in the body, eating broccoli also helps to improve and prevent a range of skin problems, particularly acne. This vegetable is also a valuable source of iron, as well as folic acid and vitamin C, making it easier for the body to absorb the mineral. For this reason, it's good for the treatment of anaemia and fatigue, and prevents birth defects such as spina bifida.

buckwheat

Most people think buckwheat is a cereal. It's actually related to rhubarb, and is suitable for anyone with gluten or wheat allergies.

It has a high content of rutin, a substance that strengthens the tiniest blood vessels, and helps frostbite, chilblains and thread veins. Anyone bruising easily or with tiny broken blood vessels under the skin should be cooking with buckwheat flour. Herbalists use extracts to treat hardening of the arteries, high blood pressure and varicose veins.

Buckwheat flour makes wonderful and health-giving pancakes, and is used for this purpose in oriental cooking. The pancakes you get with duck in a Chinese restaurant are always made from buckwheat. It's also a staple food in Russia and Poland, where it's used to make traditional tiny pancakes called blinis. Have them with a topping of smoked salmon, cream cheese or caviar (or preferably all three), and a glass of hot lemon tea if you want a truly mouth-watering experience.

butter

If you can't taste the difference between butter and margarine, there's something wrong with your taste buds. Despite the adverts, you're better off with butter. It's delicious, and in modest amounts, it's certainly healthier than nearly all margarines. It is virtually all fat and sixty percent of that is saturated fat; 100g of butter give you 740 calories, but it's a rich source of vitamins A, D and E.

Some brands are much higher in salt than others and may contain up to 1,300mg per 100g. In the UK, many brands of butter may be coloured, but they may not contain antioxidants unless the finished product is made exclusively for manufacturing or catering use, so choose unsalted, uncoloured brands.

Unlike most dairy products, butter is a poor source of calcium, but it does not contain the heart and artery-damaging trans-fats produced during the margarine-manufacturing process. Be sparing with the butter, then, and your food will taste better.

cabbage

Stir-fried, steamed, braised, stuffed or raw, cabbage is delicious. Only the great British tradition of boiling it to death renders it into a grey, sulphurous, inedible pulp. It doesn't matter what variety of cabbage you choose – Savoy, Chinese, red or white – this amazing family of plants has deservedly been known in Europe as the medicine of the poor since the Middle Ages.

Cabbage is rich in antibacterial sulphur compounds, which makes it valuable for chest infections and skin complaints like acne. It also contains healing mucilaginous substances similar to those produced by the mucous membrane of the gut and stomach for their own protection. Traditional European naturopaths used it to treat stomach ulcers. They prescribed one litre of fresh cabbage juice to be taken daily for ten days: a regime that really works.

Dark-green leaves not only contain iron but also lots of vitamin C, which helps the body absorb this essential mineral. Anyone with anaemia and all women having periods should try to eat some form of cabbage at least five times a week. In addition, it's an excellent source of folic acid, which helps prevent birth defects and contains lots of betacarotene, which is important for healthy skin.

Studies of populations show that eating lots of the cabbage-family vegetables means a much lower incidence of cancers, especially of the lung, colon, breast and uterus. It's the protective plant chemicals that produce this amazing effect, and as soon as the leaves are chopped, crushed, juiced or cooked, enzymes are released that convert these chemicals into indoles, which are anti-carcinogenic.

But there's more. As well as eating this wonderful food, you can use it externally. A large warmed, bruised cabbage leaf wrapped around a painful joint will make it feel much more comfortable, and applied to a painful breast (kept in place with a bra) will reduce the inflammation and swelling of mastitis.

caffeine

The first coffee shop opened in London in 1652; coffee consumption – and with it, caffeine – has been growing ever since. There's also caffeine in tea, chocolate and cola drinks.

On the positive side, caffeine stimulates the brain, concentration and fights fatigue. It helps some asthmatics, increases the potency of painkillers and even helps migraines. The down side is that it pushes up your blood pressure: one espresso can increase it ten percent for up to three hours. Excessive amounts cause caffeinism: tremor, irritability, insomnia and sweating. Boiled coffee increases the risk of cancer and more than three cups a day of any sort has been linked to PMS, cyclic breast lumps, poor fertility and low birth weight. Pregnant women and vegetarians should reduce their consumption, as caffeine affects absorption of the minerals iron and zinc. It also increases the amount of stomach acid produced, causing heartburn and indigestion.

So enjoy a cup of good coffee, tea or cocoa, but limit the amounts and don't get hooked.

caraway

This wonderful aromatic herb has been used in food and medicine since ancient times. The Roman cookery writer Apicius recommended it with vegetables and fish, while in medieval times it was used in bean and cabbage recipes. By the 1600s, it appeared in bread-making. Popular in European and Jewish cooking, you'll find these seeds today in breads, sauerkraut, cheeses, goulash, roast goose and cooked fruit, and as the basis for the Dutch liqueur called *Kummel*.

The medicinal value of caraway seeds is in the treatment and prevention of wind and indigestion. It's common in parts of Europe for people to chew a few seeds before a meal. Adding some seeds to bean and cabbage-based recipes reduces the 'flatulence factor'. An effective expectorant, they're a common ingredient used in children's cough medicines. Herbalists have used them for centuries as a mild diuretic and to stimulate production of breast milk. Chew the seeds for a great natural breath freshener.

carrots

Carrots contain so much betacarotene that a single large one provides enough betacarotene for your body to convert into a whole day's dose of vitamin A. Though baby carrots may taste sweeter, it's the old, dark-orange carrots that contain the most of this essential nutrient.

Betacarotene is better absorbed from cooked carrots, especially if there is some fat or oil in the same meal. We now know that, like other carotenoids, betacarotene has many vital functions of its own, most importantly in the prevention of cancer. People eating lots of carrots specifically have less risk of developing lung and breast cancer, and greater protection against many others, too.

As a powerful antioxidant food, carrots are anti-ageing and help protect the skin against sun damage and wrinkles. They're also essential in fighting arterial disease, as they help improve blood flow in the coronary arteries of the heart. Russian scientists have isolated a natural chemical in carrots called daucarine, which triggers dilation of the blood vessels and explains their circulatory benefits.

Carrots are a common traditional remedy for diarrhoea, especially puréed for children and infants. For adults with this type of problem, slice the carrots thinly, steam till tender and mix with plain boiled rice. If you've had several days of partying, clubbing, or large business lunches, and you've had too much rich food and booze, give your liver a holiday and try a two-day fast on nothing but fresh carrot juice and plenty of water to stimulate the liver.

There have been some recent scares about the high levels of pesticide residue in carrots. It is recommended that they should be peeled and the tops and bottoms discarded. Organophosphate pesticides are extremely toxic, so whenever possible, choose organically grown carrots. This is even more important if you're feeding them to babies and small children, but there are now excellent varieties of commercially available organic baby foods.

cauliflower

Like cabbage, cauliflower is a member of the *Brassica* family, and although containing the same cancer-fighting compounds, it provides less betacarotene and riboflavin. These vital constituents are easily destroyed by cooking, so cut the cauliflower into small florets, wash well and eat as a crudité with dips made from flavoured live yogurt or fromage frais.

Cauliflower is an excellent source of folic acid, which protects against heart disease and birth defects, making it a particularly healthy vegetable. It does provide some vitamin C, so it's a good immune-booster, but the white part is in fact the immature flowering head. Eating some of the tender green leaves closest to the flower will increase the amounts of vitamin C, betacarotene and folic acid that you get.

Because cauliflower is one of the very few vegetables most children will eat, serving it as cauliflower cheese provides all the benefits of the vegetable plus a huge boost of bone-building calcium many children don't get enough of.

cayenne pepper

People are always surprised about the medicinal benefits of this fiery chilli. It's a member of the *Capsicum* family, which includes all the other peppers. Cayenne has little nutritional value, but it has been used as medicine for at least 2,000 years in Asia and South America, as well as in Europe since the Middle Ages.

The most important constituent is capsaicin, a powerful circulatory stimulant. This makes cayenne an effective treatment for the relief of cold hands and feet, chilblains, Raynaud's disease and all kinds of joint pain. As well as adding it to your food, it's now available in cream form, so you can use it for external application. Alternatively, when you go for a winter walk in the cold and damp and your feet end up feeling like two blocks of ice, just sprinkle a little cayenne powder into your socks to warm them.

Make sure you wash your hands thoroughly after using cayenne, and never touch eyes or other sensitive bits with cayenne on your fingers.

celery

Because 100g of celery contains only seven calories, from a dieter's point of view it's a true 'negative food', because you burn more calories chewing, swallowing, digesting and getting rid of this plant than you get from eating it. As a vegetable, it's also a very poor source of nutrients as it's just over ninety-five percent water, although it does provide a modest amount of potassium. If you eat the unblanched, dark-green variety and the leaves, you'll also get some betacarotene and a little folic acid.

The real value of celery is its delicious flavour and powerful medicinal effects. Hippocrates, the father of modern medicine, used celery to make remedies for nervous patients – and how right he was. Essential oils extracted from the seed have a strong calming influence on the central nervous system and they also help lower blood pressure.

Wild celery was also highly valued by the Romans for its medicinal value, but cultivated varieties were developed by Italian gardeners in the Po Valley during the Middle Ages. It was only introduced to Britain as a vegetable towards the end of the seventeenth century, since when both wild and cultivated varieties have been popular with herbalists.

Celery is a traditional diuretic and helps in the elimination of water. This makes it good to eat if you have puffy hands and feet or swollen breasts just before a period. The seeds are also widely used for rheumatism, arthritis and gout, as they help remove uric acid which aggravates the pain of all these joint disorders. They're also a good antiseptic so, along with their diuretic effect, they help cystitis and other urinary infections. Put half a teaspoon of seeds in a cup of boiling water, cover and leave to steep for ten minutes, strain, add a little honey and drink three cups a day. (Don't use if you're pregnant or have kidney disease, however.)

Combine medicine and taste by sprinkling ground celery seeds into tomato juice, or mixing them with a little salt and use to flavour quails or gulls eggs.

cheese

Five thousand years ago, the Sumerians were making twenty different types of cheese, and 7,000 years before them, man was making soft cheese from sheep's and goat's milk. The ancient Greeks and Romans were great cheese-makers and their products were highly valued as an important food. In fact, every Roman legionnaire was entitled to a daily portion of cheese. So why, in the twenty-first century, are we turning our backs on this amazing source of pleasure and essential nutrients?

I grow increasingly concerned that many people, especially young women, interpret a low-fat diet as being a no-fat diet, and for this reason exclude most dairy products from their regular food intake. Sadly, this is not always done for health reasons; it's much more likely to be in the pursuit of thinness.

As a source of calcium, for building strong bones; essential protein; vitamin D, to help absorb the calcium; a selection of B vitamins for the central nervous system; vitamin A as a cancer-fighter; and for healthy skin and a spread of essential minerals, it's hard to better an ounce of good cheese.

Cheese supplies some zinc in an easily absorbed form, and 100g has a quarter of your daily needs. Zinc is vital for normal male sexual function. Cheese is also good for children and adolescents, as they need the calcium for their bones. Worryingly, around half of British youngsters don't get enough.

Some people with migraine react badly to the chemical tyramine in cheese, which can trigger attacks; there are also those with an allergy to cows milk. Goat and sheep cheeses make a wonderful alternative, and for both of these groups, they usually present no problems. Most goat cheese is soft and mild, but if you like hard cheese, then the Spanish sheeps' milk Manchega is exceptional: hard, with a full but mild flavour. French Roquefort, Italian Pecorino and Greek feta are among the more strongly flavoured sheep cheeses.

cherries

Is there anything that tastes better than the first cherries of the season, especially as they're one of the few seasonal fruits only available for a few months of the year? It may be convenient to have other fruits and vegetables in the supermarkets 365 days a year, but the best nutritional content comes from fruits and vegetables eaten in season, grown as close to where you live as possible and harvested in peak condition.

Cherries probably came originally from the orchards of Mesopotamia in pre-biblical times, and were certainly highly valued by the ancient Greek physicians. They are a fairly recent arrival in Europe, introduced as the wild cherry from Asia, and though most wild fruits are quite bitter, the wild cherry is sweet and succulent. Of the cultivated varieties, my favourites come from the orchards of Kent. Most cherries in supermarkets are imported.

Of the sour cherries, morello are wonderful for cooking, bottling, juicing and liqueurs, and the acerola is the richest in nutrients, especially bioflavonoids. Wild cherry bark was used medicinally, and the dried fruit stalks and fruits are an effective diuretic. Cherries contain plenty of potassium and virtually no sodium, so they're excellent for anyone with high blood pressure or heart disease.

They're a reasonable source of vitamin C but they also contain significant amounts of bioflavonoids and other plant chemicals, which make them pretty near the top of the list of protective antioxidant foods. It is the ellagic acid content that adds extra value to their anti-cancer properties.

In folk medicine, cherries have been used for the relief of arthritis and gout, and dried cherry stones make the most wonderful hot bag for muscular pain, joint disorders and stomach-ache.

chestnuts

Apart from stuffing the turkey at Christmas and maybe roasting a few on the fire, chestnuts are a much under-used and underrated food. As far back as prehistoric times they were eaten by the earliest hunter-gatherers, and to this day they are still regarded as staple foods in some parts of the world, particularly in southern Italy.

Unfortunately, they produce poor crops in Britain and they must not be confused with the poisonous horse chestnut used by herbalists. They must be cooked first, but you can then add them to sweet and savoury dishes, vegetables, soups or stuffings. Try cooking a few with Brussels sprouts or adding them to broccoli-and-Stilton soup.

Unlike most other nuts, chestnuts contain virtually no fat and only 170 calories per 100g. Because they're high in starch, they can be dried and ground into excellent gluten-free flour. There's not much protein, but they do contain B vitamins, thiamine (B_1), riboflavin (B_2), pyridoxine (B_6) and potassium.

chickpeas

Chickpeas, like all the pulses, are an amazing food. They're cheap, filling, versatile, easy to use and delicious. You can buy them canned, whole, split or ground into flour.

If you're using dried beans, they need to be soaked in cold water for six hours, then rinsed well before cooking. Canned chickpeas are already cooked and ready to eat, but they must be strained and rinsed thoroughly to remove the salt. Add canned chickpeas to recipes at the end of cooking; otherwise they turn into mush.

Never add salt when cooking chickpeas, as this toughens the skins and makes them more difficult to digest; it's best to season them after cooking. They're great in soups, stews and casseroles and extremely popular in Middle Eastern cooking, where they are the basic ingredient of hummus and falafel. This pulse has a unique savoury, nutty flavour and nutritionally provides protein, manganese, iron, folic acid and vitamin E.

chocolate

Feeling low and a bit depressed? Eat some dark chocolate. It's delicious and is there to be enjoyed, so ignore the 'food police' who say it's unhealthy. Good-quality chocolate is, in fact, a source of valuable nutrients as well as pleasure.

The Aztecs were the first to discover chocolate, and the cocoa tree was originally native to Mexico. In earliest times, it was so highly prized that the Aztecs used the cocoa beans as currency; only members of the royal family were allowed to consume it as a drink.

When making chocolate, most of the fat is left in and the quality is determined by the percentage of cocoa solids in the finished product. Most British chocolate is made with added milk, but on the Continent the taste is for much darker forms with a higher percentage of cocoa solids. The very best chocolate contains a minimum of seventy percent.

When the famous botanist Linnaeus named the cocoa tree, he called it *theobroma*, meaning 'food of the gods'. A major constituent of the bean is theobromine, which triggers the release of natural 'feel-good' chemicals in the brain. It's these endorphins which help depression and kindle the feelings of romance, love and arousal. Caffeine is also present, which helps make chocolate a mild diuretic.

Herbalists have used chocolate for its theobromine and the stimulating effect on the heart muscle and the kidneys. Chocolate was traditionally used, combined with *Digitalis*, for fluid retention linked to heart failure, and because it dilates the blood vessels, it can also be useful in the treatment of high blood pressure.

Although it contains fat, dark chocolate is a very good source of iron and magnesium. Chocolate supplies useful amounts of protein and traces of other minerals and some B vitamins. But it's loaded with calories: over 500 per 100g. You'll need to walk briskly for two hours, pedal your bicycle for an hour and a half, or swim nonstop for an hour to burn off 100g of chocolate.

cranberries

Cranberries are native to North America, and for centuries the American Indians have used them for food and medicine. They washed injuries in cranberry juice, and their medicine men made cranberry poultices to draw poison from arrow wounds. It was the Indians who helped the pilgrims survive by teaching them to live off the land. Thanks to the high vitamin C content in cranberries, they avoided scurvy, and it wasn't long before American whalers were carrying barrels of cranberries, just as the English sailors used limes.

American folk medicine has long prescribed cranberry juice to relieve cystitis, and modern science has now proved the truth of this ancient knowledge. Originally, doctors thought it was the acidity of the juice that killed off the bugs but this is not the most important mechanism. Cranberries contain substances that stick to the lining of the bladder, kidneys and internal plumbing, and they stop bacteria making their home in these sensitive tissues. One glass of cranberry juice is ten times more effective than antibiotics. Most importantly, chronic sufferers should continue with their daily glass even after symptoms have disappeared, as this is a powerful preventer of recurrent attacks.

There are pure organic juices on the market, but do be careful with the more commercial brands as many of them contain low levels of juice and far too much sugar or artificial sweeteners; it's important to read the labels. If you're drinking pure juice, dilute it fifty/fifty with water and do not brush your teeth within half an hour of drinking. This applies to any acidic fruit juice, as the acid softens tooth enamel which is then easily damaged by brushing.

When the Native Americans introduced those early starving settlers to the wild turkey, Indian corn (maize), squash, sweet potatoes and cranberries, they saved their lives. To this day Americans celebrate Thanksgiving with a meal of turkey, cornbread, sweet potatoes, pumpkin pie and of course, cranberry sauce.

dandelion

Traditional English folklore warns children about what happens if they pick dandelions; the north country name for this extremely valuable medicinal plant is 'wet-the-bed'. In France, where you buy it by the kilo in any street market, it's known as *pis en lit* – for the same very good reasons.

Both leaves and roots of the dandelion have historically been used as a diuretic and in the treatment of gall bladder and liver problems ever since the Middle Ages. The leaves help constipation and are good to eat in pregnancy.

It's the bitter taste of the leaves that gives the clue to their value, as it is the unique natural ingredients that stimulate the liver and the production of bile, which in turn improves fat digestion. The leaves are rich in vitamins A and C, as well as iron.

So leave them in the garden and use young leaves tossed in extra-virgin olive oil with bits of crispy bacon: a traditional French salad for fatigue, skin or joint problems.

dates

Dates have been a vital food crop for 5,000 years, and although they don't contain much in the way of vitamins, they're a rich source of minerals and instant energy. Their iron content, which is little appreciated outside of the East, varies according to variety, but most contain highly significant amounts in an easily absorbed form. You only need ten Gondela dates from the Sudan or fourteen Khidri from Riyadh to provide your daily requirements.

This high iron content, together with the easily available energy, makes dates an excellent nutrient for those suffering from anaemia and illnesses which produce chronic fatigue. Bearing in mind the desert-roaming Bedouin often travelled for days with little more to eat than a store of dates, figs and flour to make their unleavened bread, why not add a few to the lunch-box, for child or adult, instead of a bag of sweets? As a bonus, throughout the Middle East, dates are believed to be an aphrodisiac.

dill

Never plant dill too close to fennel, as they're so closely related that you may end up with a hybrid and lose this herb's distinctive flavours. The frond-like leaves add a wonderful flavour to salads, fish, eggs and most vegetables. The seeds have a less pungent smell but a much stronger taste, and they are the traditional addition to pickled cucumbers. They're also excellent added to salad oils and vinegars – especially the cider and wine varieties – as they seem to enhance their natural taste.

Dill contains the volatile oils carvone, limonene and phellandrine, and it's these that make them extremely effective in the relief of flatulence, stomach pain and indigestion. Use the leaves or seeds to make a tea for rapid relief.

Herbalists have long recommended dill to help stimulate the flow of breast milk in nursing mothers, and most babies taste it in gripe water. No coincidence, then, that its name comes from an ancient Saxon word meaning 'to lull'.

duck ·

Duck meat is an excellent source of protein, iron, zinc and nearly all the B vitamins. Be warned, though: delicious as the crispy skin is, you will get 29g of fat if you eat 100g of meat and skin, but only 9.7g if you stick to the meat alone. Like chicken, it's even more important to cook duck on a rack. It also helps to prick the skin all over with a sharp fork or skewer, so the fat layer under the skin can trickle out as it melts in the heat of the oven. Served with the traditional apple sauce, it not only tastes wonderful, but the pectins in the apple helps the body eliminate much of the cholesterol eaten with the duck.

Commercially reared birds, like the famous Aylesbury duck, are widely available, but if you ever get the chance to eat the wild fowl, take it. The flavour is slightly stronger, but the fat content is much, much less.

eggs

Eggs are the ultimate protein. Ninety percent is utilized by the body, compared with only sixty-seven percent from steak and thirty percent from lentils. They're also a wonderful source of zinc and vitamins A, B, D and E.

One of the most important substances in egg yolk is lecithin, which is vital as part of many of the body's metabolic processes, including the dispersal of dangerous fat deposits and cholesterol. Lecithin prevents the development of heart disease as well as the formation of gallstones, and also encourages speedy conversion of body fats into energy.

Because of their high lecithin content, eggs are an important brain food, contributing not only to memory and concentration, but also to good mental and emotional status.

Modern man's obsession with cholesterol means that people have drastically cut down on the number of eggs they eat and go to ridiculous lengths like making disgusting omelettes from one whole egg and three egg whites. Yet there is a big difference between dietary cholesterol and blood cholesterol. The body manufactures cholesterol when you eat saturated animal fats, but the cholesterol in eggs *does not add* to the circulating blood levels; it is only a factor in people who already have extremely high cholesterol or suffer from hereditary diseases which mean they make too much of their own.

You'll be happy to know that the World Health Organization advises a maximum of ten eggs a week. Factory-farmed battery eggs should be avoided as they are much more likely to be infected with salmonella and contain chemical additives that are added to the feed. Always choose organic hens eggs.

Duck and goose eggs are also delicious, but they need to be thoroughly cooked. Hard-boiled quails eggs with a little celery salt are also a wonderful treat. If you want the ultimate 'eggstacy', try gulls eggs for the most delicious, creamy-textured yolks.

fennel

Fennel has been used by the Greeks, Romans, Anglo-Saxons and the American Puritans. It was a diet aid for Roman women, while the Puritans nibbled a handful of seeds to stave off hunger during their extremely long church services.

Tea made from the crushed seeds is a good expectorant for coughs and bronchitis, and this herb also relieves flatulence, improves digestion and stimulates the liver. Fennel is a useful diuretic, and an infusion of the seeds is helpful for kidney stones and cystitis.

Seventeenth-century herbalists recognized fennel's value as both food and medicine, and it has long been used to flavour all kinds of fish dishes. Most fennel is grown for its feathery leaves and seeds, yet the stately bronze fennel is one of the most beautiful plants in the herb garden.

Florence fennel produces a large white bulb that is delicious when eaten raw in salads or cooked, as its aniseed flavour is sweeter than the wild fennel.

figs

If Adam and Eve used fig leaves, they must have eaten the figs – and I never understood why they bothered with the apple. There are many other biblical references to figs, both as food and medicine. Isaiah, for example, told King Hezekiah to apply a fig poultice when he developed a tumour.

Figs do indeed contain the anti-cancer agent benzaldehyde, as well as healing enzymes, flavonoids and a particular natural chemical, ficin, which starts the breakdown of proteins and improves digestion. Figs are a rich source of iron, potassium, betacarotene, fibre and energy, and throughout Asia are revered as one of the most aphrodisiac of foods.

Buddhists, Hindus and even the Romans regard the fig as a sacred tree, and extracts of the fruit, leaves and bark are important in Indian Ayurvedic medicine. The earliest Olympians consumed masses of fresh figs for strength and stamina. Either fresh or dried, they provide instant energy, potassium to ward off cramp and lots of healthy fibre for modern athletes.

fish

Tragically, the consumption of fish has been declining for years – which is bad news nutritionally, as fish is one of the healthiest of all foods. It's also perfect for slimmers, which makes it even more extraordinary that in a time when obesity is on the increase and dieting is a national obsession, we still manage to eat less and less of the fruits of the sea.

White fish and most freshwater fish, with the exception of salmon, trout and eels, are a terrific source of protein and minerals and virtually no fat. They provide lots of B vitamins, but their flesh contains virtually no vitamin A, D or E. Fish roe will give you as much iron as the same weight of pork chops or roast lamb.

The oily varieties are another kettle of fish as, thanks to the fats they contain, they provide much more energy and much more of the fat-soluble vitamins. Anchovies, whitebait, herring (see page 64), sardines (see page 96), sprats, mackerel, pilchards and tuna contain vital amounts of omega-3 fatty acids which are essential for normal cell function, powerful anti-inflammatories and vital to the growth and development of the brain and central nervous system during pregnancy and breastfeeding. Yet again, folklore is proved correct – when grannie said eat fish for your brains, she was right.

These oily fish are a vitally important source of vitamin D, without which the body cannot absorb calcium. It's these cheap and quick-to-cook foods that prevent rickets in children and osteoporosis in adults. Two to three portions of oily fish a week are really essential during pregnancy, and an enormous health bonus at all other times. Few people get enough iodine in their diets, essential for the thyroid gland to regulate metabolism. Sea fish is the best of all sources.

Read labels on cans and avoid 'vegetable oil' as this mixture certainly contains saturated fat from palm oil. Olive and sunflower are best.

garlic

Garlic was brought to Britain by Roman centurions who wedged fresh cloves between their toes to prevent foot rot. Some of the discarded garlic took root and this wonderful wild plant soon became established.

Some years ago, a strange coincidence turned me into a garlic freak. Three patients told me their doctors were puzzled by changes in their blood samples. They'd all come to me with different conditions, but the one thing they had in common was heart and circulatory problems, for which they'd been prescribed anticoagulants to 'thin' their blood. In the same week their doctors had reduced the dose of their medication because their blood was getting too thin.

Why did I find this news so exciting? Because the only common treatment that I prescribed for all of them was large doses of garlic.

From as far back as ancient Egypt to Greece, Rome, England in the Middle Ages, and up to the end of the nineteenth century, garlic was the most widely used medicinal plant in the world. Bronchitis, catarrh, sore throats, asthma, indigestion, constipation, diarrhoea and even athlete's foot can all be helped by this powerful little bulb. But by far the most exciting development in the history of this plant is research into its heart and circulatory benefits. In countries where it's eaten in abundance, fewer people die of heart attacks than in the UK and America.

The sulphur compound allicin, released when garlic is crushed, both encourages the elimination of cholesterol from the body, and reduces the quantity of the unhealthy fats which are produced by the liver. In healthy volunteers on fatty diets it has been shown to reduce the level of cholesterol in the blood by up to fifteen percent. Another experiment showed that patients with high cholesterol levels who were given garlic tablets but no dietary advice reduced their cholesterol by twelve percent in four months.

ginger

Ginger is a warming, antiseptic spice widely used in meat and fish cooking in the East. In the West, it's also a popular sweet spice used dried with fruits like melon, preserved to make rhubarb and ginger jam, and crystallized as confectionery. It has been used since 5,000 BC in India and China as both a culinary and medicinal plant. In Indian Ayurvedic medicine, it is considered one of the most important remedies, and traditional Chinese herbalists use some of the non-edible forms for the relief of arthritis, rheumatism and other inflammatory pains. Even the Roman Apicius included ginger in many of his recipes for sweet and savoury sauces.

This wonderful root contains zingiberene, gingerols and very pungent shogaols. Dried ginger contains a higher proportion of these substances, which is why it's much sharper and, to my taste, less palatable than the fresh root. Ginger is the best of all remedies for the prevention of travel sickness and early morning sickness in pregnancy. It's not only completely safe for children, mothers-to-be and the baby in the womb, but clinical trials have shown that it works even better than the normal prescription drugs.

It's effective against coughs, colds, bronchitis and sore throats, and half an inch of fresh ginger grated into hot water, lemon juice and honey as a bedtime drink is a perfect treatment for a cold. As a nausea remedy, you can buy ginger tea-bags, but making your own tastes better and is very simple. Peel and grate half an inch of ginger root into a cup. Add boiling water, cover and stand for ten minutes. Strain, add a teaspoon of honey and sip slowly. For colds, flu or simply to ginger up body and mind, just add the juice of half a lemon.

Most exciting of all are the latest American studies which show that ginger extracts are just as good for the treatment of arthritis as the standard anti-inflammatory drugs – without any of their dangerous side effects.

grapefruit

As the perfect eye-opening, wake-up food, grapefruit must be top of the list. Whether you like the sharp, tart taste of ordinary grapefruit or prefer the sweeter, more succulent flavours of pink grapefruit, the benefits are the same. Like all citrus fruits, they are an extremely rich source of vitamin C, and half a grapefruit or a glass of juice will give you enough for the whole day. Grapefruit has become such an important food that it supplies the average American with sixty percent of the daily requirement of vitamin C.

They're also a good source of potassium and bioflavonoids, both important for your heart and circulation. The soluble fibre pectin is another valuable ingredient which helps the elimination of cholesterol from the body. Pink grapefruit is a good source of a number of the strongly antioxidant carotenoids which help protect against heart disease and cancer, including betacarotene, which the body converts into vitamin A – essential for skin, the mucous membranes and the natural defence mechanisms.

But not everyone should start their day with this delicious fruit. If you're taking a particular type of the special heart and blood-pressure pills known as 'calcium blockers', then you shouldn't take grapefruit or its juice less than a couple of hours before or five hours after your medication.

Drugs (like cyclosporin) which suppress the immune system, which are used for very severe rheumatoid arthritis, kidney disease, severe psoriasis and after transplant surgery may also react badly with grapefruit. If you're not sure, read the leaflet that comes with your medicines or check with your doctor.

If you only drink the juice or prepare your fruit so that you eat the flesh and leave the dividing skin and pith behind, you're missing out. It's these parts that are richest in pectin and bioflavonoids. Why not peel the grapefruit and eat the segments like an orange, making sure you leave plenty of the pith attached?

grapes

Grapes contain an enormous number of aromatic compounds – far more than all other fruits. Most important of these from the health point of view are the astringent tannins, flavones, red anthocyanins, linalool, geraniol and nerol. These powerful antioxidants are what make grapes such good all-round protectors against heart and circulatory diseases as well as cancer.

Since the earliest times, grapes have been used to produce wine and raisins. Vines were first taken to the New World by Columbus in 1492, then again by the Spanish and Portuguese, who took them to South America. Wine was an essential part of the Communion ritual, so vineyards were important.

It's no accident that these succulent fruits are what most people take to friends in hospital. They are uniquely nourishing, and help in the treatment of anaemia, fatigue, arthritis, gout, rheumatism and especially in convalescence and recovery from surgery or serious illness. Always wash grapes thoroughly in warm running water to remove pesticide and herbicide residue.

guava

If you want a taste of heaven, put a carton of natural bio-yogurt, a fresh peeled guava and 200ml of semi-skimmed milk into a blender and whiz until smooth. Rich in calcium, gut-friendly bacteria, vitamins and fibre, this is a real powerhouse addition to any breakfast.

The guava, a relative of cinnamon, cloves, allspice and nutmeg, is an extremely good source of vitamin C and can contain up to 400mg in 100g of fruit – a week's worth. It's best to eat guavas slightly underripe, as they lose vitamin C if you leave them to ripen too much. They also supply plenty of fibre, some phosphorous and calcium, as well as B vitamins.

Guava juice is one of the most delicious drinks around, but you will need to make your own as the commercially available ones are nearly always 'nectars': a mixture of twenty-five percent fruit, ten percent sugar, and sixty-five percent water.

herring

Herrings are a member of the *Pelagic* species of fish, and like their relatives mackerel, pilchards, sardines and sprats, they're known as fatty or oily fish. Up to twenty percent of their weight are fats of the healthiest kind, making them a wonderful source of polyunsaturated and other long-chain essential fatty acids. These have a strong anti-inflammatory effect, are totally essential for brain and nervous-system development in babies and can dramatically reduce the risks of strokes and heart disease.

Around sixteen percent of their weight is protein, they're rich in the fat-soluble vitamins A, D and E, and they're a good source of water-soluble B vitamins. Add to all this a good spread of minerals and you can understand why herrings are such an important food. It's a real tragedy that these cheap, delicious and easy-to-cook fish seem not to appeal to today's shoppers, especially when you compare their nutritional benefits with ready meals, take-aways and the ever-growing junk food market.

In Victorian times, the average Londoner consumed 7kg of herring a year and an average of four oysters a week, these being foods for the poor, just like the cockles and whelks which they also ate in huge quantities. In the early twentieth century, however, most Britons preferred white fish – and it was then that lack of vitamin D and atmospheric pollution (which blotted out the sun's rays) caused a major epidemic of the bone disease rickets; vitamin D is essential for the body's ability to absorb calcium and turn it into strong bones. Jewish children in London's East End seldom got this crippling disease, due to their taste for pickled, salted and fresh herrings.

Like all the oily fish, herrings must be eaten very fresh, as they are extremely perishable. Turning herring into kippers by smoking them stops the fat becoming rancid, gives them a much longer shelf life and a wonderful flavour. Choose undyed kippers and you will avoid any toxic chemicals.

honey

Honey is a good example of getting what you pay for. Mass-produced, blended, imported honey is cheap, has very little flavour and bears little resemblance to the wonderful produce of the individual beekeeper who knows where his bees collect their nectar.

Ancient societies throughout the world used honey as an energy food, for sweetening, and as a preservative, and the combination of milk and honey has religious connotations in many civilizations. It's referred to in the Old Testament, was frequently used as an offering to the gods by Romans, and Greeks, and to this day is a popular bedtime drink for insomniacs.

Honey contains fructose, glucose and sucrose, and lesser amounts of maltose and dextrins: all forms of sugar. Thanks to its fructose content, however, honey is much sweeter and contains fewer calories than cane or beet sugar. If you must sweeten tea and coffee, use honey for fewer calories and more flavour. It also contains an amazing substance called propolis: a natural antibacterial produced by the bees to protect the hive from infections. That's why real honey never grows mould or goes off.

For thousands of years, honey has been used for medicinal purposes: both internally as a hot, soothing drink for coughs, colds and the relief of stomach pain, indigestion and ulcers, and externally to heal wounds, cuts and abrasions. Plastic surgeons apply it to reduce scarring after surgery, and it is traditionally used to treat leg ulcers. Modern research has investigated the properties of Manuka honey, long used by Maori tribesmen in New Zealand for stomach complaints and wound-healing. This is now known to be so powerfully antibacterial that eating it kills the *Helicobacter pylori* bug that causes stomach ulcers. And it's even effective against the dreaded hospital infection MRSA, where most antibiotics fail. Naturally produced, unfiltered honey contains pollen grains, which is why it's an effective treatment for hay fever. Eat honey from local hives; the bees feed on the plants that trigger your allergies. Three dessertspoons a day can have a dramatic effect.

horseradish

Today horseradish is a popular condiment, but it has been cultivated for centuries as a medicinal herb. Pliny advised it exclusively as a medicine, and biblically it's one of the five bitter herbs that Jews eat during the celebration of Passover. The powerful antibacterial and anti-cancer properties come from its natural content of siligrin, which breaks down to form isothiocyanates. The plant is rich in sulphur, and its traditional English use as a condiment with roast meats and oily fish is an aid to their digestion.

This powerful root is a wonderful remedy for coughs and sinus problems; it very quickly encourages expectoration and makes the eyes and nose run, clearing the sinuses within minutes. A teaspoon of fresh, grated root with a teaspoon of honey in a cup of boiling water is a remedy for sore throats, blocked sinuses and flu, and an old wives' treatment for hay fever is a sandwich of freshly sliced horseradish – only for the brave.

kale

Kale is a member of the cabbage family and is grown for its shoots and curly, greenish-yellow leaves. It almost certainly started life in Western Europe, but it is now distributed throughout the world. With all the anti-cancer properties of the cabbage family and a huge amount of betacarotene – 100g provides almost a whole day's dose for the average woman – we should all be eating far more of this delicious vegetable.

Because it is much less bitter than dark-green leafy cabbages or spring greens, it's the perfect vegetable to use to encourage children to eat their greens. Kale is also one of the best sources of lutein, one of the carotenoids that specifically helps prevent an eye disease called Age-related Macular Degeneration (AMD), the most common cause of visual loss in the elderly.

One of the great traditional dishes of the hardy Dutch is *Stumpot*: a delicious mixture of mashed potato mixed with lightly steamed and chopped kale with meat or sausage and gravy.

kiwi fruit

These fabulous, furry fruits used to be called Chinese Gooseberries, but then New Zealand farmers perfected them as a commercial crop – and they're now the world's major producer. They renamed it kiwi fruit, after the country's national emblem, the kiwi.

Kiwi fruit contains almost twice as much vitamin C as oranges and more fibre than apples. Just one provides twice as much vitamin C as you need for a day and, unusually, the vitamin C in kiwi fruit is extremely stable. Inevitably there is a decline immediately after picking, but even after six months, ninety percent of the vitamin C is still there.

Kiwi fruit is a good boost to the immune system, is helpful for nearly all skin problems and it's a good aid to the digestion. It really is a wonderful food for children, and I've found that the best way of encouraging youngsters to eat them is to put one in an egg cup, slice off the top and let them eat it with a spoon, just like a boiled egg.

The high potassium content of kiwi fruit is extremely important, as most Western diets are very high in sodium (seventy-five percent comes from processed foods) and very short of potassium. Potassium deficiency and sodium excesses are a major cause of high blood pressure, strokes and heart disease. Just missing out on potassium can affect the heart muscle, cause muscle cramp during exercise and can also be a factor in insomnia, exhaustion and depression. An average kiwi fruit will give you around 250mg of potassium, but only about 4mg of sodium.

The fibre content of kiwi fruit and the particular type of mucilage it contains make it an excellent but extremely gentle laxative. They also contain a digestive enzyme called actinidin: similar in action to the papain in papaya. It helps in the breakdown of animal protein and is a useful addition to marinades as it tenderizes meat before cooking. Kiwi fruit is perfect for the elderly, who seldom get enough vitamin C and frequently suffer chronic constipation.

leeks

Leeks are a member of the all-powerful *Allium* family – garlic, onions, chives – and though not as rich in the anti-carcinogenic chemicals, they, too, are important in the detoxification process. They are also antibacterial and, as such, contribute to the protection against stomach cancer, destroying some of the bacteria in the gut that change harmless nitrates into cancer-causing nitrites.

Leeks have been cultivated for at least 4,000 years as both food and medicine. Ancient Egypt was once described as a country in which 'onions are adored and leeks are gods'. The Greeks and Romans held them in the highest esteem, especially for the treatment of throat and voice problems. The infamous Emperor Nero ate leeks every day to improve the quality of his singing voice, and in French folk medicine, leek soup was a traditional prescription for all breathing problems.

Famous throughout the world for their male-voice choirs, the Welsh adopted the leek as their national emblem, and they're worn by Welshmen and -women throughout the world on St David's Day. Was it, I wonder, only done to celebrate the historic triumph of their king, Cadwallader, when the Welsh defeated the Saxons in 690 AD (the Celtic soldiers wore leeks so they could recognize friends from foes)? Or was it perhaps to improve the quality of their battle songs?

Although leeks contain only small amounts of vitamins, minerals and fibre, they are a reasonable source of folic acid and vitamin C, and a good source of potassium. They are diuretic and have the ability to eliminate uric acid, so they are an excellent food for anyone suffering from gout or arthritis.

When preparing leeks, most people discard the dark-green leafy parts that normally grow above ground and eat only the white stem. This is a great mistake, because the green bits are a good source of betacarotene, which the body converts into vitamin A.

lemon balm

Lemon balm (also known as melissa) was used in Greek medicine as long as 2,000 years ago. Traditionally, it was planted near beehives and in orchards, as bees are always attracted to the fragrant flowers. Herbalists have used it for depression since the Middle Ages, and it's used for the same reason today by aromatherapists.

Made into a tea, it's a remedy for anxiety, tension, stress and insomnia, and it's great for kids, too. Throughout Spain, lemon balm is every mother's cure-all for her children's headaches, tummy troubles and temperatures. Modern research shows that lemon balm is antiviral and helps heal cold sores. Simply dab them with a strong infusion of the leaves, or crush a leaf in your fingers and rub it gently on the sore; this also works for insect bites and stings.

It smells wonderful but tastes awful when cooked, so add fresh leaves to salads or fish dishes at the end of cooking.

lentils

Like all pulses, lentils contain lots of protein and valuable amounts of B vitamins, together with iron, zinc and calcium, though the minerals are not well-absorbed unless you eat vitamin C-rich foods at the same meal.

Indian vegetarians always eat rice or Indian bread with dhal. This combination of cereals and pulses provides all the essential amino acids needed for the body to get complete protein. Lentils are also a rich source of fibre, so they prevent constipation, help lower cholesterol and protect against bowel cancer. If you're stressed, exhausted or both, the B vitamins, especially niacin, make them a perfect nerve food. If you've got gout, however, be careful, as lentils contain purines, which will aggravate the condition.

Unlike other pulses, there's no need to soak lentils before cooking. And although there are different varieties, the nutritional value is the same whether they're red, yellow, green or brown.

liver

The ancient Persian writings contained in the *Ebers Papyrus*, the oldest surviving prescription book, contain a treatment for night-blindness. Simply roast an ox liver over the fire, grind it to a paste and administer to the patient who has problems seeing in the dark. This prescription would certainly have worked dramatically well, as night blindness is caused by deficiency of vitamin A, though I'm sure the ancient Persians weren't aware of this.

Liver is lovely and an amazing source of essential nutrients – but try telling that to the children. Liver pâté or sausage are both quite high in saturated fat, but I've always found it easier to get children to eat these a couple of times a month, as the benefits far outweigh the fats.

Liver is an abundant source of well-absorbed iron (essential for healthy blood) and zinc, which is vital for active sperm and a healthy prostate gland. Lack of iron is a common cause of anaemia, especially in women, and zinc deficiency results in loss of appetite and chronic fatigue.

Liver is also the richest of all sources of vitamin A and vitamin B_{12}. In the mid-twentieth century, injections of ox liver, which contains the most B_{12}, were the only treatment for pernicious anaemia. All animal livers are an excellent source of vitamin A, which you need for night vision, natural immunity, protection of all the mucous membranes and for healthy skin. On top of all this, it contains important quantities of riboflavin, pyridoxine and folic acid.

health warning

If you're pregnant or even trying to get pregnant, DO NOT EAT ANY liver, liver pâté or liver sausage. When I was a student, all pregnant women were advised to eat liver once a week, but now we know that, although sufficient vitamin A is essential for the baby's development, excessive amounts ingested during pregnancy can cause serious birth defects. One teaspoonful of lambs liver contains a day's dose of vitamin A, while an average portion of liver gives you over 500 percent.

maize

Mexico is believed to be the original native home to maize. This crop, also called corn, is now the second-largest cereal crop in the world, and apart from Antarctica, it grows virtually everywhere. It is the staple food in many of the world's most deprived areas. It's a cheap and reliable provider of energy-giving calories as it needs only a short growing season, produces a high yield and can survive in areas of extremely low rainfall.

Unfortunately, maize does not contain the natural chemical tryptophan, without which the body is unable to absorb nicotinic acid, one of the B vitamins. This is the reason that the deficiency disease pellagra occurs in populations who depend mainly on maize as their staple food, who consume little or no milk and very little or no animal protein. Though scientists knew about nicotinic acid in 1840, it was 100 years before the link was made between this B vitamin and pellagra, a disease that killed 2,000 Americans in 1940.

The name pellagra comes from the Italian *pella* for skin and *agra* meaning rough. In this condition, after the early symptoms of weight loss, weakness and mental difficulties, the skin becomes itchy and scaly, especially on the hands, face and neck. Sores in the mouth and tongue, dementia and problems with the brain and nervous system follow. If the condition is treated before irreversible damage is done to the nervous system, the symptoms improve within a day of taking the first dose of nicotinic acid. In spite of understanding the causes, there are still outbreaks of pellagra in parts of Africa and India. In the West, it's mostly alcoholics who suffer with this disease.

Maize is converted into many different products: cornflakes, popcorn, cornflour, polenta, grits, and even corn syrup, used as a sweetener. It's a gluten-free cereal, so it's fine for anyone with Coeliac disease, for whom Mexican tortillas and all other maize products are suitable.

mango

An average mango provides more than a day's dose of vitamin C, two-thirds of vitamin A, nearly half vitamin E, almost a quarter of fibre, and useful amounts of potassium, iron and nicotinic acid. It also tastes wonderful, so it's not surprising that it's probably the most eaten of all tropical fruits. A native of India, its history goes back more than 4,000 years. Today, varieties are grown in Australia, South Africa, and Brazil, but my favourite is the small, sweet fruit from Pakistan.

It's a bonus that anything tasting this good is so healthy and a source of extremely powerful, protective antioxidants. Mangos are medicinal as well; in traditional Indian medicine, the antiseptic twigs are chewed to protect teeth and gums, the bark for the treatment of diarrhoea and the fruit for high blood pressure.

Mangos belong to the same family as poison ivy, so if you're preparing lots of them, wear gloves to avoid contact with the potentially very irritating skin.

millet

Because millet is never highly refined, it retains all of its essential nutrients. It can be used as a thickener in soups, stews and vegetable casseroles, or it can be ground into a coarse flour and used to make a biscuit-like bread. There are many different varieties of millet, but this is a much-ignored cereal in Britain and the US, although it is popular with 'food reformers'. It should be much more widely used.

This easily digested cereal is gluten-free, so it is suitable for anyone suffering from coeliac disease. It's high in protein, low in starch and particularly rich in the mineral silica. This essential nutrient is a prime ingredient of collagen, the body's glue that binds everything together, and is needed for healthy hair, skin, teeth, eyes and nails. This high-quality, protein-rich grain is a perfect food for children and invalids, or for anyone who is convalescing after an illness or operation.

mint

No one should ever need to buy this wonderful herb as it grows anywhere. If you put it in the garden, use a bucket with drainage holes sunk into the ground; otherwise it takes over. It'll grow happily in a pot, and both leaves and flowers are wonderful to eat.

There are many different varieties of mint, each with it's own distinctive flavour. If you have space grow several, especially *Mentha spicata* (spearmint), *Mentha spicata Moroccan* (the perfect variety for tea), as well as ginger and pineapple-flavoured varieties.

Spearmint is the oldest medicinal variety, as well as being the common garden mint; it's best for sauce with roast lamb. It has an ancient history stretching back to the Roman Empire, where it was used as a tonic and mental stimulant, and legionnaires took it with them, like garlic, throughout the world. The Egyptians left sprigs of it in the pharaohs' tombs. It's also mentioned in the Bible, and the Japanese have been extracting its essential oils since the first century.

Mint tea is a simple treatment for stress-induced headaches. Chewing the leaves or drinking the tea stimulates the cortex of the brain to improve concentration and creates feelings of inner peace and harmony.

Yet it's as a digestive aid that mint comes into its own, which is why its culinary use with fatty meat like lamb is so popular. Mint improves fat digestion and is an effective antacid, thanks to the essential oils menthol and menthone, flavonoids and menthyl acetate. Peppermint oil is still the basis for many prescribed and proprietary indigestion remedies because it is extremely soothing to the stomach lining. Because it relaxes the muscles of the digestive tract, it helps relieve irritable bowel syndrome, stomach cramp and general indigestion.

All over the Middle East, meals end with a glass of mint tea for digestion. To make your own, simply tear up half a dozen mint leaves into a glass, add boiling water, cover, stand for five minutes, sip and enjoy.

mushrooms

Thousands of years ago, the Egyptians believed mushrooms were a gift from the god Osiris. Ancient Romans said they resulted from lightning thrown to earth by Jupiter during storms; this explained their sudden appearance, as if by magic. The Chinese wrote about mushrooms in the Chow Dynasty 3,000 years ago, explaining how they were used as both food and medicine. Other evidence suggests man was using them 4,000 years earlier than that.

We should all eat more mushrooms. They contain more protein than most other vegetables, are very low in calories, and are good sources of phosphorous and potassium. Although most of the textbooks state that mushrooms are not a source of vitamin B_{12}, the most up-to-date research reveals they are a valuable source of this essential nutrient. One decent-sized field mushroom (or three button mushrooms) will give you enough B_{12} for a day – vital for vegetarians and even more so for vegans, as other plant sources of B_{12} are very limited. The same is true for vitamin E, which is listed as zero in most textbooks. Again, modern research reveals that most mushrooms are a rich source of this essential nutrient: 100g provides more than the minimum daily requirement.

Mushrooms and truffles are the edible portions of fungi; mushrooms appear above ground, truffles below. Of course, not all mushrooms are edible. Some are very poisonous and others taste revolting. Dried mushrooms generally have a much fuller flavour; although expensive, many Italian, Japanese, Chinese and French varieties are now widely available. For modern food researchers, Japanese and Chinese mushrooms are medicinally interesting. Shiitake boosts immunity, for example, Reishi is good for liver disease, high blood pressure and asthma, and Maitake for blood pressure, liver disease and boosting immunity. Washing spoils their delicate flesh, so brush away any grit and wipe clean with a damp cloth.

nutmeg

All those wonderful Victorian nannies were very clever, and I'm sure it was no accident that rice pudding was a favourite nursery dish. Traditional recipes always included a good sprinkle of nutmeg: the ancient herbalist's equivalent of a modern 'happy pill'. Rice pudding at lunch meant an easy afternoon for the nannies.

Nutmeg and mace both come from the same plant, an evergreen tree called *Myristica fragrans*, which is native to the Indonesian Molucca Islands. Nutmeg is the inside of the seed, while mace is the dried outer covering of the shell.

As far back as the sixth century nutmeg was an important part of the spice trade and widely used in India and the Middle East. Extremely popular in Holland, it's added to everything from cabbage and stews to sweet desserts. The Dutch took it to South Africa, and to this day pumpkin cooked with honey and nutmeg is served with savoury dishes.

The smell and taste of nutmeg and mace are similar, though mace has a slightly more bitter flavour. The most important chemical in nutmeg is myristicin, which has a profound effect on the brain and is chemically similar to mescaline, derived from the famous peyote cactus in Mexico. Nutmeg also stimulates the appetite and is a valuable digestive remedy for food poisoning, diarrhoea and nausea. In India it's used as an aphrodisiac, especially for men.

The hallucinogenic properties of nutmeg are extremely powerful; prisoners on the chain gangs in the southern states of America used to smuggle nutmegs back into the prison and used them as narcotics to make them feel happy. In small doses nutmeg and mace are perfectly safe, but there are reports of death resulting from consuming two whole nutmegs.

This is also an important spice in Indian Ayurvedic medicine, where it's added to traditional remedies for insomnia, coughs and nausea and believed to promote healthy skin.

oats

Get your oats – and make sure you do it every day as they're one of the most important of all cereals. They have a high nutritional value, providing good amounts of protein, heart-protective polyunsaturated fats, B vitamins and vitamin E, combined with calcium, potassium and magnesium. They're one of the best foods to nourish the nervous system, as well as building strong bones and teeth.

From ancient 'kitchen medicine' to the twenty-first century, oats have been valuable as both food and medicine. They're a highly effective treatment for depression, and herbalists use tinctures of the plant to help patients overcome addiction to tranquillizers.

The soluble fibre in oat bran helps the body get rid of bile acids that would otherwise be converted into cholesterol. Reductions of up to twenty percent have been measured in patients given a daily dose. It's this same fibre that makes porridge, or oats in any form, the best treatment for even the most chronic constipation. Unlike wheat bran, which can sometimes be an irritant, oat bran works more like 'smoothage' than roughage. Oats have the added advantage of not interfering with mineral absorption, as they do not contain phytic acid.

Oats also have a vital role to play in the active prevention of adult onset diabetes – a condition we are now seeing in growing numbers of young children. Oats have a low glycaemic index (GI), which means they release sugar very slowly into the bloodstream; this reduces the production of insulin and the consequent risk of developing diabetes.

As if all that weren't enough, few people realize how good oats are for the skin. Four tablespoons tied into a muslin bag, soaked in the bath and used as a sponge are healing and soothing for dry skin, eczema and psoriasis. This amount is enough for four or five baths. You can even buy oat-based creams and ointments for local application.

olive oil

How the world has changed. When I was a student, the only place to find olive oil in the UK was at the chemist's, who sold it in tiny bottles for dropping into ears. Thank goodness you're now spoiled for choice in every supermarket, deli and corner shop. Olive oil is the basis of the Mediterranean diet, which we know dramatically reduces the risks of heart disease, high blood pressure, strokes and many forms of cancer.

Extra-virgin olive oil is expensive, but it is the best and should be used for salads, dipping your bread in, and grilling delicately flavoured foods such as fish. Virgin olive oil is slightly more processed, and regular olive oil may be both heat and chemically treated. Which country's oil you choose depends entirely on personal taste. It's really worth experimenting to find which you like the best.

Using olive oil avoids the consumption of saturated animal fats but it also has its own specific health benefits. The mono-unsaturated fats in the oil help reduce cholesterol levels, and because of its high vitamin E content as well, the oil acts as a strong antioxidant, protecting every individual cell from damage. But there are other benefits, too. Some of the natural chemicals in olive oil prevent the absorption of cholesterol and increase the level of what are called HDLs: high-density lipoproteins. It's these that remove the artery-clogging and dangerous LDLs (low-density lipoproteins) from the bloodstream.

Olive oil is the best-digested of all the vegetable oils and produces the most effective stimulation of the gall bladder. This is important for overall fat digestion, as the bile stored in the gall bladder breaks down fatty foods into tiny droplets, which are then more easily processed by the digestive juices. This makes olive oil not only valuable for the relief of liver and gall-bladder problems, but also one of the most important things you can eat to protect your liver.

onions

Onions belong to the same family as garlic, leeks, spring onions, chives and shallots, and not only do they taste good, they do you good as well. We all love our fried egg and bacon breakfast, and in one of my favourite experiments it was given to a group of volunteers. Half of them also got a portion of fried onions. Blood tests then measured the clotting tendency of both groups. Without the onions, there was increased risk of clotting, with them a reduced one. So if you fancy a fry-up, make sure you don't forget the onions.

Wild onions are a traditional medicine of native North Americans for the treatment of colds, stings and bites. Chinese herbalists use them as a poultice for boils, and in European folk medicine they've been used for anaemia, bronchitis and asthma, genito-urinary infections, arthritis and rheumatism, gout, and premature ageing. A night on the tiles in Paris traditionally ends with a steaming bowl of onion soup to prevent the next day's hangover. In East Anglia, thick onion soup was a favourite for treating chesty children.

Onions contain the enzyme allinase, which is released when you slice the bulb. The action of allinase on sulphur compounds in the flesh results in the chemicals that not only give onions their flavour but also make you cry. They're very low in calories, but spring onions especially are a good source of vitamin C, as well as small amounts of some B vitamins and traces of minerals.

Onions are diuretic, both dissolving and eliminating urea, which makes them useful in the treatment of rheumatism, arthritis and gout. Like all their relatives, they are also strong antibacterials.

Onions can even help your chilblains. Simply rub the affected area with a thick slice of raw onion. If you've got a colicky baby, put a few slices of onion in a jug of hot water, strain after five minutes and, when cool, give the baby a teaspoonful.

papaya (pawpaw)

This delicious and nutritious tropical fruit was originally a native of southern Mexico and Costa Rica. Taken to Manila by sixteenth-century Spaniards, it's now grown throughout the tropics. Today, most of the world's supplies come from the United States, where papaya are grown in abundance in Hawaii.

Nutritionally, the papaya is very important in developing countries, as it fruits year-round and is rich in vitamin C. Papaya is also an excellent source of betacarotene, which the body converts to vitamin A. One fruit will give you twice your requirement of vitamin C and almost a third of vitamin A, so papayas boost immunity and are good for the skin and mucus membranes.

Their most important constituent is an enzyme known as papain, which improves digestion. This natural chemical is extracted and dried to a powder that is used by industry as a meat tenderizer. Traditional medicine men of the South American Mayans used the sticky latex, the juice and fruit as herbal medicines, and it's still common in South America to wrap meat in papaya leaves before cooking to produce tender and delicious dishes.

The leaves are also used to improve wound healing, leg ulcers and for the treatment of boils in traditional medicine. And even the seeds are useful. Next time you eat one, save the seeds and add them to olive oil, vinegar and pickles for a unique and very different spicy flavour.

Pawpaws are wonderful for children and make great-tasting smoothies. Halve and deseed the fruit, scoop the flesh into a blender, add a small carton of yogurt and a cup of milk and whiz until smooth and creamy. For adults, whiz with a little water and mix half-and-half with Champagne.

Canned papaya is widely available, but it is nutritionally poor compared to the fresh fruit. Most of the vitamin C and more than half the betacarotene are lost during the processing.

paprika

Paprika is one of the most important traded spices. It's a product of the *Capsicum annuum*, which began life, like all the peppers, in South America. The most famous use of paprika is in Hungarian cooking, where it's the prime ingredient of goulash, traditionally the beef soup of Hungarian cowboys – not the thick stew more popular today. Quite how this particular capsicum arrived in the Balkans is actually a bit of a mystery, but they probably came with the travelling Turks during the seventeenth century. The plant was soon established in Hungary, where the warm summers encouraged the development of the wonderful aroma produced by the essential oils in the plant.

The Hungarians and all the Balkan countries use large amounts of paprika for both colour and flavour. It's rich in carotenoids and contains capsaicin, a circulatory stimulant – though not as much as the hot South American chillies. These capsicums are often seen growing in Spain but seldom in the rest of the Mediterranean.

parsley

The Greeks and Romans loved parsley. They used it as a diuretic and a digestive, and it's valued for the same properties today. Rich in essential oils, coumarins and flavonoids, it also supplies vitamin A and C, some iron, calcium and potassium.

Juiced with apple, carrot and celery, it's an ideal breakfast drink for women suffering monthly fluid retention. It's also delicious and nutritious added generously to all salads.

It's easy to make your own parsley tea. Put a large handful of chopped leaves into a jug, add 850ml of boiling water, cover, leave for ten minutes and strain. When cool, keep it in the refrigerator and drink a glass every three hours as a gentle, natural diuretic.

If there's parsley on your plate, don't push it to one side. Eat it, especially if you've got arthritis, rheumatism or gout, as it aids the elimination of uric acid. Chewing a sprig also freshens the breath after onions, garlic, or too much alcohol.

parsnips

Parsnips are a prime example of foods that should be eaten in season. The modern supermarket trend to have all foods available from the four corners of the earth throughout the year means that over-cultivated, forced and artificially fed produce ends up on the plate with very little flavour and, almost certainly, diminished nutritional value.

This much-ignored and often denigrated vegetable deserves to be treated much better than it is. It has a unique and delicious flavour and can be used in far more interesting ways than just throwing a few cubes of soggy vegetable into a pot of stew, soup or casserole.

The Romans knew a thing or two about food, taste and health, and had magnificent kitchen gardens attached to their villas. The emperor Tiberius ordered regular supplies of fresh parsnips to be sent from the banks of the River Rhine to Rome.

The wild parsnip has been used for centuries in Europe, where it grows around the borders of cultivated fields and in chalky soil in roadside verges. Like carrots, they've long been a popular cultivated vegetable with a history of countryside use. In Germany, they're often eaten together with salted fish during Lent; in Holland, they're used for soup; in Ireland, they were boiled with water and hops to make beer; and English countrywomen turned them into jam and parsnip wine.

The herbalists Culpepper, Gerard and Tournefort, and even evangelist John Wesley, were all fans of the humble parsnip and advised it for both humans and livestock. How right they were, as parsnips provide calories, fibre, potassium, folic acid, vitamin E and traces of minerals and other B vitamins.

They taste best after the first hard frosts of winter. Mash them together with swede, carrot or potato, or brush with a little olive oil and roast. They're even fabulous cooked on the barbecue.

pasta

Pasta provides complex carbohydrates for slow-release energy, and while wholemeal varieties contain more fibre, minerals and B vitamins, both white and wholemeal are healthy. The idea that pasta is fattening is one of the longest-surviving food myths; it's what you put on it that makes the difference. A creamy carbonara sauce with bits of fatty bacon; bolognaise made from high-fat mince; lasagne that is more cheese than pasta... all of these are certainly high in calories. But the classic *aglio e olio* – spaghetti with garlic and olive oil – or a simple mixture of extra-virgin olive oil, garlic, parsley, rosemary, thyme and basil (*spaghetti alle erbe*), or a dish of pasta with tuna fish and spring onions are all wonderful meals: filling, satisfying, delicious and a weight-watcher's delight.

Like sun-dried fruits and vegetables, cured, smoked or air-dried fish and meat, pasta is one of the oldest convenience foods. Once made and dried, it can be kept for months and cooked in minutes.

Traditional Italian pasta divides into simple basic categories:

Pasta lunga (long pasta)	spaghetti, spaghettini, angel hair, linguini, fusilli etc.
Fettucce (ribbons)	tagliatelli, fettuccini, tagliolini, etc.
Tubi (tubes)	such as penne, macaroni, rigatoni
Odd shapes	like farfalle, conchiglie, orecchiette, lumache, fusilli
Stuffed pastas	ravioli, cappelletti, tortelloni, canneloni, lasagne, etc.

Marco Polo brought pasta home to Italy from China in 1295. It's made with flour milled from durum wheat, which has a high gluten content, making the dough so elastic. In spite of the popularity of fresh pasta, often made using egg and a softer flour, serious Italian cooks tend to prefer dried pasta for the majority of recipes. Today, there are quite palatable wholemeal varieties available, even in supermarkets.

peaches

Many food books describe peaches and nectarines as different varieties of the same fruit, nectarines sometimes being dubbed as 'smooth-skinned' peaches. In fact, nectarines are no more than a genetic variation of the peach, and both are part of the *Prunus* family of prunes, plums and apricots. The botanical name for the species is *persica*, because early botanists thought they started life in Persia. It's more likely that peaches first grew in China and were introduced to Persia by early traders.

Peaches and nectarines are now grown commercially all over the world, wherever the climate is suitable. Italy and Spain are the biggest European growers, and vast crops come from America. Commercial peaches are heavily sprayed, so buy organic when you can; otherwise, wash them (and all other fruit) thoroughly before eating.

Nutritionally, neither peaches nor nectarines are really great sources of any single nutrient, and there is little difference between them. Both contain good amounts of vitamin C, nectarines slightly more: one will give you a whole day's requirement. A little fibre, some betacarotene and small amounts of minerals are also available, but because they are virtually salt- and fat-free, they're ideal food for anyone with raised cholesterol and high blood pressure. Best of all, they're low in calories and smell and taste fabulous.

Dried peaches contain far more calories, but 100g will provide almost a day's requirement of iron and a third of your daily need for potassium. Canned peaches may taste good, but they are nutritionally poor, as most of the vitamin C has gone and they're often canned in syrup that is so very high in calories.

In addition to the benefits of this wonderful fruit, peach leaves are a great home treatment for boils. Soak in boiling water till pliable, press out any surplus water and, when cool enough not to scald, apply as a poultice to the boil and cover with a clean cloth.

peanuts

I can hear you all throwing up your hands in horror and saying, 'This man's mad! What on earth are peanuts doing in a book on healthy eating?' Well, I'm telling you the truth about this wonderful and highly nutritious food. When I ask my patients if they like peanut butter, most of them hang their heads in shame and whisper, 'Yes…' as if it were their guiltiest secret, because almost every woman I know believes that peanuts – and even worse, peanut butter – are guaranteed to pile on the pounds. The facts, however, reveal the exact opposite.

Over the last two or three years, scientists have proved that the common low-fat diet is not nearly as effective for weight loss, nor does it protect against heart disease as well as the Mediterranean concept of a moderate-fat diet which consists mostly of vegetable fats and oils. Most recently, a large-scale experiment demonstrated that eating a teaspoon of peanut butter five days a week helped the participants to lose, on average, a pound a week.

What's more, the mono-unsaturated fats in peanuts reduce cholesterol levels and protect against clogged arteries and heart disease. Additional benefits come from the high content of fibre, folic acid, vitamin E, potassium and the amino acid arginine, which is crucial to heart health.

Peanuts are also one of the great preventers of adult-onset diabetes as they have a super-low glycaemic index, which means they hardly raise blood-sugar levels so that the body doesn't need to pump out lots of insulin. All this protection, prolonged energy release, and a wonderful source of nutrients mean that peanuts and peanut butter should be part of your regular eating pattern – as long as you're not allergic to them, and as long as you choose the plain or dry-roasted varieties over their more greasy and salty counterparts.

pears

Most people think of pears as something you occasionally stick in the fruit bowl. But this is a serious mistake because, although they contain very small amounts of essential nutrients, they have other health-giving properties which are extremely valuable.

Pear trees are native to Europe, and many of the popular modern varieties were propagated by Belgian and French gardeners during the 1700s. My favourite, 'Conference', first grew in Berkshire, but Williams, Red Williams, Comice and Packham are all popular varieties of this delicious fruit.

Pears are a good source of the soluble fibre pectin, which not only helps regular bowel function, but also increases the amount of cholesterol eliminated by the body. They're a reasonable source of vitamin C, some vitamin A and E, and useful amounts of potassium. For digestive problems or convalescence, pears are an easily digestible source of good calories. There's no fat, virtually no sodium and the fruit sugar is easily converted into energy.

Pears are one of the foods least likely to cause any type of allergic reaction, so they're ideal puréed for babies, and used in exclusion diets where food allergies or intolerances are suspected. However, fresh pears do contain a sugar-based alcohol called sorbitol. While this sugar-free sweetener is tooth-friendly, in large amounts it may cause diarrhoea in a small number of susceptible people.

Like all dried fruits, the nutritional value of dried pears is much higher than that of the fresh fruit. They have a very high natural sugar content, which makes them a perfect high-energy snack to sustain you during the day, and to provide the necessary energy before and after physical activities. They also have high levels of potassium, which also helps prevent cramp during exercise, and they contain significant amounts of iron. Drying increases the vitamin A content, and though some vitamin C is lost, some remains in the fruit, together with high levels of natural soluble fibre.

peas

The average Brit eats more peas than any other vegetable apart from potatoes, making them the most popular of vegetables. Sadly, a large proportion of these are canned, and though whole canned peas retain some nutrients, canned processed peas – usually mushy peas – lose almost all their vitamin B and C. To make matters worse, both processed varieties have high levels of salt.

Fresh green peas provide an excellent source of thiamine (vitamin B_1); 150g supply more than a day's need. They're also a good source of folic acid, and supply useful amounts of vitamin A and C. Peas are a good source of protein, but they need to be combined with cereals such as rice, pasta or bread to make complete protein.

All forms of peas and chickpeas are excellent sources of fibre. Because the sugars in peas start to convert into starches as soon as the pods are picked from the vine, many people prefer the sweeter taste of frozen peas, though nothing matches the wonderful flavour of home-grown peas straight from the garden.

Modern technology allows peas to be frozen almost instantly after harvesting, conserving both their sweetness and most of their vitamin C content, and they can be kept frozen for up to a year without nutritional losses. Dried peas and chickpeas are also nutritionally valuable but don't contain any vitamin C. Sugar-snap or mange tout have the same sort of nutritional value as green peas, but because you eat the whole pod, you get considerably more of the vitamins A and C.

Vitamin B and vitamin C are destroyed by heat, so when cooking fresh peas, only boil them long enough to just soften the texture and make sure you use the cooking water in gravies, stocks or soups. Frozen peas have already lost some of their nutrients, so cook them in the minimum amount of water for as short a time as possible – otherwise, the losses become quite significant.

peppers

Sweet peppers are a terrific source of vitamin C, providing between 60mg and 170mg per 100g of flesh, depending on colour. The colour changes as the fruits ripen, starting at green, the lowest vitamin C level, and ending as red when fully ripe, with almost three times as much of this essential nutrient. Red and yellow varieties also provide considerable amounts of betacarotene. Weight for weight, even a green pepper will give you twice as much vitamin C as an orange, and more than your minimum daily requirement.

Peppers are very low in calories (around fifteen per 100g) contain no fat and virtually no sodium. They do supply folic acid, potassium and fibre, making a valuable contribution to the diet. As well as the betacarotene, they're an excellent source of bioflavonoids; both these substances are powerful protective antioxidants which increase the body's defences against degenerative diseases such as arthritis, cancers, and heart and circulatory diseases. They also play a major role in the prevention of age-related macular degeneration (AMD), the most common cause of visual impairment in the elderly. This is because peppers contain the special carotenoids lutein and zeaxanthine, nutrients which don't occur that widely in nature but specifically protect the tissues of the eye.

An added benefit of peppers is that the waxy substances in their skin prevent oxygen passing through into the flesh, thus protecting the fruits against damaging oxidation which also destroys vitamin C. Unlike almost every other variety of fresh produce, their vitamin C content remains very high even weeks after harvesting – even more so if they're kept refrigerated.

Peppers, like pimentos and chillies, belong to the *Capsicum* family, which originated in the Americas. Columbus brought them back to Europe, and from there they spread to Africa and Asia. Native Americans have used this whole family of plants for more than 5,000 years both as food and, in the case of chillies, as medicines, too.

pineapple

'Apart from vitamin C and few calories, there's very little to recommend pineapple.' How wrong can you be! This sweet, delicious tropical fruit has been a healing food since earliest times. Sore throats, digestive problems, blood clots and bruising all respond to some of its natural ingredients, with the added benefit of pineapples being both antibacterial and anti-inflammatory.

In the early 1900s, boxing trainers gave their fighters fresh pineapple before each contest. They were very clever, as they knew it reduced the amount of bruising, keeping their boxers looking their best.

The benefits are due to a natural enzyme called bromelain, which can break down many times its own weight of protein in just a few minutes. Happily, it only attacks dead and damaged tissue so doesn't interfere with the lining of the stomach and digestive tract. There are several hundred published research papers about the benefits of pineapple, showing that it is helpful in dispersing blood clots, attacks the bacteria that cause urinary infections and sinus problems, and may actually increase the effects of antibiotics.

Bromelain has also been shown to be an effective anti-inflammatory, making it an exceptionally good fruit for anyone with arthritis, both osteo and rheumatoid. If you're an active sportsperson, pineapple should always be a regular on your shopping list, as it helps stimulate the body's repair mechanisms, thus helping to heal strains and sprains.

You will only get the benefits from ripe pineapples, and uniquely, they stop ripening at the moment of harvest; after that, they just rot. Pulling the leaves out of the top is an old wives' myth – the only way to judge ripeness is by weight, and if the fruit feels heavy for its size, it's full of sweet juice and ready to eat. Soft pineapples will be brown and fermented, and unripe ones will never be improved by sitting in your fruit bowl. Only the fresh fruit and the juice contain beneficial bromelain.

potatoes

Let's get this straight once and for all: potatoes are *not* fattening; it's what you do to them that makes the difference. One hundred grams of boiled potatoes contain only eighty calories. Roast them and it's 157 calories; turn them into chips and its nearly 300, and crisps give you 533 calories from just three bags. Potatoes were the staple food of the Irish for generations, and they supply fibre, B complex vitamins, minerals and vitamin C. Eating the skin is a bonus, as it contains potassium and other nutrients, too. First cultivated by the Incas of South America, who gave the world corn as well as the potato, it's certain that the Spanish took potatoes into southern Europe, but it was Sir Francis Drake who introduced them to both Ireland and Britain.

The starch in cooked potato is easily digestible, so it's good for invalids, anyone with digestive problems and particularly as a weaning food for infants. The biological value of potato protein is just as good as the soya bean; one large jacket potato provides a quarter of your daily need and also over half your vitamin C requirements for a day. In fact, potatoes account for around half of all the vitamin C in the average UK diet – which is a sad reflection on how little fruit and vegetables we consume.

Naturopaths have traditionally used raw potato juice as a highly successful treatment for stomach ulcers and osteoarthritis. It's simple to do: drink half a small wineglass of the juice four times a day for a month. The taste is vile, but you can camouflage it by adding apple and carrot juice, or some honey. Alternatively, add the fresh juice to any soup just before you eat it, but not during cooking.

If you've got high blood pressure, drink a mug of potato-peel tea every day, as it contains lots of potassium. If they're not organic, scrub thoroughly and add a dessertspoon of coarsely chopped peel to a mug of boiling water. Never use green skin or flesh – they're poisonous.

poultry

Poultry embraces domesticated fowl such as chicken and farm-raised turkeys, geese and ducks (see separate entry, page 56). Until the days of factory farming chicken and turkey were seen as luxuries and kept mostly for special occasions, Christmas and Thanksgiving. Though wild duck and goose were favourites with the hunters, domesticated versions were still expensive.

Chicken and turkey are now so cheap that they're everyday foods for most people, but the price we pay is the lack of flavour and texture, a higher saturated-fat content and the risk of unwanted chemical residues such as antibiotics and growth-promoting hormones. For your health, and especially that of your children, buy organic. It is more expensive but eat it less often and you won't feel the pinch.

The domestic chicken descends from the Indian jungle fowl and was certainly eaten by the ancient Egyptians by the fourteenth century BC. Chicken contains less fat than red meats; most of it is in the skin and easily removed. In addition to protein, chicken provides easily absorbed iron and zinc – twice as much in the dark meat as the breast, but the breast has double the B_6, which fights against PMS. Before roasting, remove all fat from the body cavity and cook on a rack to allow the fat to drip through.

Goose contains huge amounts of iron, zinc and vitamin B_{12}, but nearly as much fat as protein. To cook, place it on a rack over a large pan of water. Cover with foil, making sure it's tucked inside the pan. Bring to the boil and steam the bird for half an hour, which removes a lot of fat. Then roast on the rack, deducting half an hour from cooking time. Delicious though it is, don't eat the skin.

Turkey, on the other hand, is extremely low in fat, and rich in protein, iron and zinc. Traditional free-range birds have much better flavour and texture, and you can enjoy the low-fat crispy skin.

Never throw away any poultry leftovers as they all make fantastic and nourishing soups which are rich in vitamins, minerals and healing enzymes.

prawns

Prawns belong to the family of crustaceans that includes shrimp, crab, lobster, crayfish and scampi, and real prawns are native to our chilly island waters. Most of the frozen prawns on the market are imported, and their size varies from the small English prawn to the larger Dublin Bay prawn and Italian scampi, through to the big Pacific prawns and the enormous varieties that come from icy Scandinavian waters.

Whichever you choose, they're an excellent source of protein, vitamins and minerals, and they're extremely healthy. Unfortunately, these crustaceans have had a bad press in recent years, because they contain cholesterol. Many doctors and nutritionists advise against them or suggest they should be eaten infrequently and in small quantities. For those of you who love these seafoods, I'm delighted to say that you can relax and enjoy them with pleasure and gusto. They do contain cholesterol, but it is very poorly absorbed during digestion, and they do not contain any of the saturated fats which the body then converts into the cholesterol that's ready to clog up your arteries. There are many published nutritional studies which show that eating prawns actually *reduces* the amount of cholesterol in the bloodstream.

How you cook them makes a huge difference, of course. Boiled prawns contain 107 calories per 100g, whereas fried scampi has 316. Boiled, they contain only 1.8g of fat, which rockets to 17.6g when they're fried.

Like all seafood, prawns have a high sodium content, so never add salt when cooking or eating them. Prawns are a really good source of vitamin B_{12}, which makes them an important food for those who do not eat meat but are happy to consume fish. They also supply iodine, a mineral often lacking in the UK diet and which is essential for the proper function of your thyroid gland, and calcium for strong bones. They're an excellent supplier of selenium – essential for a healthy heart and protection against prostate and breast cancers.

prunes

How dreadfully maligned these wonderful dried fruits are. In countries like France, where food is so much appreciated, they're considered a delicacy, whereas we tend to consider them for one purpose only – and that's the least of their value.

Prunes are the dried fruit of a variety of plum which grows around the French town of Agen, below Bordeaux. The Crusaders brought them to Britain from the Middle East, but it was the Arabs who planted them in France much earlier. *Pruneaux d'Agen* is the name unique to this area, and they are as strictly controlled as any fine-wine *appellation contrôlée*.

In the twenty-first century, seventy percent of the total world supply of prunes comes from sunny California, which produces twice the crop of the rest of the world put together. It is fascinating that this now-huge Californian industry began when California nurseryman Louis Pellier persuaded his brother to bring cuttings of the prune plums from Agen back to California after his marriage in France in 1856.

Prunes are rich in potassium, making them valuable for those with high blood pressure. They're also rich in fibre and iron and contain useful amounts of niacin, vitamin B$_6$ and vitamin A. They're an excellent source of energy, as they are so easily digested and produce 160 calories per 100g. Prunes also contain a chemical called hydroxy-phenylisatin, which stimulates the smooth muscle of the large bowel; it is precisely this characteristic that makes them an effective, gentle, non-purging laxative.

Most importantly of all, weight for weight, prunes are the most powerful of all the protective antioxidant foods. The US Department of Agriculture has calculated the Oxygen Radical Absorbance Capacity, or ORAC, value – a measure of the protective value of foods – at 5,770 units per 100g, compared with 2,000 for raisins, blueberries and blackberries, and 980 for a plateful of Brussels sprouts. A handful of prunes provides the optimum protection of 5,000 ORACS a day.

radishes

Radishes are part of the *Cruciferae* family, like cabbage, broccoli and Brussels sprouts, and as such they contain glucosilinates and other sulphurous compounds that are valuable for those at risk from cancer. But it is for gall-bladder and liver problems that herbalists have found this delicious vegetable most useful. Radish juice has a powerful effect on the gall-bladder, making it contract and pump more bile into the stomach. It's this increase in bile that improves the digestion of fats, which is probably why radishes are so popular in France as a pre-dinner nibble. If you've never tried the traditional French snack of hot radishes dipped in butter, then salt, you've missed a wonderful treat.

Radishes are a rich source of other nutrients, too, as they contain potassium, calcium, sulphur, vitamin C, folic acid and selenium. But you can have too much of a good thing, and eating a whole bunch of radishes could irritate the liver, kidneys and gall bladder. For some people, the hot, peppery flavours can be a problem, and anyone with ulcers or gastric inflammation should treat them with caution. Like most of the *Cruciferae*, radishes can be affect the thyroid gland, and shouldn't be eaten by anyone with thyroid problems.

In the time of the pharaohs, radishes were regarded as a valuable food source – so much so that workers building the pyramids were paid in garlic, onions and radishes. In traditional Chinese medicine, they were listed in medical texts towards the middle of the seventh century. Although originally native to southern Asia, they're now widely cultivated throughout Europe, Britain, China and Japan. Surprisingly, they didn't reach the UK until the mid-1500s, when they were listed in an early herbal and recommended for their diuretic action and the prevention of gallstones.

Eat them as fresh as possible, while they're still young and crisp. And by the way, don't throw away the green tops; they're delicious and equally nutritious.

raisins

The best-quality raisins and those with the most succulent flavour are produced from grapes which are allowed to dry naturally in the sun while still on the vine. In commercial production, they're laid out in bunches on the earth for about three weeks and turned regularly till they're dry. Australia and California are the major producers of raisins, and in both places they're dried in open-sided sheds to protect them against extremes of weather.

All the nutritional benefits of grapes are concentrated into raisins, making them a wonderful store of instant energy. Just 100g of raisins contain almost 70g of the natural sugars glucose and fructose. This makes them the perfect energy food for active people. Raisins are also ideal for anyone suffering from tiredness and exhaustion for any reason, whether it's anaemia, overwork, lack of sleep or chronic fatigue.

Unlike sweets and sugary drinks, they're rich in all sorts of other nutrients: fibre to help reduce cholesterol levels and improve bowel function; iron, with 100g providing more than twenty-five percent of the RDA for women; selenium; and a huge amount of potassium, which prevents fluid retention and helps reduce blood pressure. Raisins also contain small amounts of vitamin A and the B vitamins. The combination of available energy and B vitamins means that raisins are helpful for anyone with depression, anxiety, stress and nervous tension.

Man has been drying fruits in the sun as a way of preservation for at least 5,000 years, and the Romans in particular included raisins in many of their medical prescriptions. When early settlers first travelled to the US, they took their dried fruits with them; today, raisins are firmly established as an American favourite. Many of the very finest raisins, especially the natural Thompson seedless, are now produced in California.

Organic raisins may not look so good, but aren't treated with sulphur or mineral oil. Both can be removed by washing in warm water.

rosemary

In classical Greece, rosemary was revered as a remedy for depression and despondency, and its reputation was richly deserved. It is a true food for the mind and spirit – a perfect tonic for anyone who feels 'one degree under'.

Valued for its powers of 'remembrance', rosemary is both a tonic and stimulant of the brain's cortex. It eases general debility, improves memory loss, and reduces nervous tension. Modern research shows that it increases the amount of oxygen that individual cells are able to absorb, thus improving cell function and efficiency – which explains its effect on memory.

Originally a native of the Mediterranean, rosemary is a herb surrounded by myths and legends and highly favoured by mystics, magicians, old wives and sacred healers. One fable says that a rosemary bush will grow for thirty-three years and then die – as Christ did in his thirty-third year. Elizabethan couples carried rosemary on their wedding day as a sign of fidelity, and its fragrance was believed to ward off diseases like the plague.

Scientifically, the essential oils contained in rosemary are what provide many of its medicinal benefits. Borneol, linalool, esters and tannins are just some of the constituents which give it its antifungal and antibacterial properties. Rosemary tea makes a breath-freshening mouthwash, while the oil relieves joint pain and headaches as well as being a good insect repellent.

Used with lamb and chicken dishes throughout the Mediterranean, rosemary also contains camphor, limonene and rosemaricene; this is the reason it's anti-inflammatory. It also stimulates the gall bladder to increase the flow of bile to aiding fat digestion. In addition, the rosemaricene is a mild painkiller.

As a real treat, try hanging a bunch of rosemary sprigs under the hot tap of your bath to make the water truly invigorating and reviving to both body and spirit.

sage

Sage is one of the cleansing, antiseptic and anti-inflammatory plant used by herbalists for menstrual problems, sweating and chest infections. Red sage, a Chinese relative, contains tanshinones, substances that stimulate the coronary circulation. It's also a powerful antiseptic, so try a teaspoon of chopped red sage in a glass of boiling water, cover it for ten minutes, and strain and cool before use.

Thujone is a phytoestrogen which helps to regulate periods and relieves many unpleasant menopausal symptoms, especially hot flushes. Because of its hormonal action, don't eat too much sage if you're breastfeeding, as it can reduce the flow of milk.

Its proper name is *salvia*, from the Latin *salvere*, which colloquially means 'to be in good health'. It's great with rich meats such as pork and venison, and is wonderful in the classic Italian dish of calves liver with sage. It's another herbal aid to fat digestion. If stung or bitten by insects, rub the area with a few crushed sage leaves to relieve pain.

sardines

Fresh sardines cooked on a barbecue with a bowl of salad, a glass of wine and a chunk of real bread is a royal feast almost everyone enjoys on a Mediterranean holiday but hardly ever cooks at home. Fresh sardines are cheap to buy and widely available – even in supermarkets. They're rich in protein, iron and zinc, and are a very important source of vitamin D – without which you can't absorb calcium and build strong bones. Like all oily fish, sardines supply the essential omega-3 fatty acids needed for proper development of the brain and all other nervous tissue.

Canned sardines are just as nutritious and have the added bonus of providing lots of calcium as, weight for weight, they're the only food which supplies more of this bone-building mineral than milk. That is, as long as you eat the bones. Mashed up with some Worcestershire sauce, balsamic vinegar and a squeeze of lemon juice and eaten with hot toast and a ripe tomato, they're a brain-, bone- and body-building feast.

spinach

Spinach is exceptionally rich in folic acid, which is easily absorbed; 100g provides three-quarters of the adult daily requirement. This should put spinach firmly on the shopping list of every woman planning pregnancy or already expecting.

Cancer patients or those at risk from cancer, such as heavy smokers, should also eat lots of spinach. Cancer research has shown that spinach contains even more of the protective carotenoids than other dark-green or brightly coloured fruits and vegetables – even carrots (they may be rich in betacarotene, but not the other carotenoids). Two of these special chemicals, lutein and zeaxanthine, are major protectors of your eyesight, and spinach is one of the richest sources of both. The most common cause of impaired vision and blindness is age-related macular degeneration (AMD), and American studies have shown that people who regularly consume spinach and collard greens are much less likely to develop this debilitating illness than those who don't.

As every Popeye fan knows, spinach is rich in iron. But sadly, in this respect, generations of mothers who've tried forcing spinach down their children's throats have largely been wasting their time. The substantial amounts of iron and calcium in spinach are not easily available to the body, as spinach also contains oxalic acid. This combines with minerals that are excreted as insoluble salts. As spinach also contains uric acid, anyone with gout or arthritis should eat it sparingly.

This is an extremely versatile vegetable. The baby leaves can be eaten raw in salads; it makes an ideal snack just wilted for a few minutes and served with a little butter topped with a poached egg, or cooked without the addition of water, allowed to cool and served just warm, sprinkled with finely chopped raw onion, a squeeze of lemon juice, a dash of olive oil and a sprinkle of ground nutmeg.

strawberries

There is a popular myth that anyone with arthritis should avoid strawberries because they are acidic; however, nothing could be further from the truth. In fact, strawberries are probably the nicest treatment you can imagine for this painful joint condition. These succulent fruits have an amazing ability to increase the body's elimination of uric acid: a substance that is highly irritating to inflamed joints.

Until the early 1600s, the only strawberries available in the UK and Europe were the tiny but succulent wild strawberry. Originally alpines, they were greatly valued as a delicacy and as a medicine. All the other strawberries that we enjoy today are descended from two American varieties.

Strawberries contain modest amounts of iron, but because of their extremely high vitamin C content, this is well-absorbed, which also makes them a good remedy for anaemia and exhaustion; 100g of strawberries provides almost twice your daily requirement of vitamin C.

Strawberries are an excellent source of pectin, a soluble fibre that helps eliminate cholesterol. Together with their high content of antioxidants, this makes strawberries a valuable weapon against heart and circulatory disease as well as a remedy for anyone already suffering from these diseases. There is also evidence of antiviral properties.

This is one medicine that doesn't need a spoonful of sugar to help it down. These wonderful berries should be eaten on their own, or at the start of a meal in order to achieve their therapeutic best. A daily bowl of strawberries is the cheapest and most delicious health insurance you'll ever buy.

Instead of sugar and cream, try adding a sprinkle of freshly ground black pepper. It may sound peculiar, but the heat of the pepper seems to draw out maximum flavour from the berries. If you want to be really adventurous, add a spoonful of balsamic vinegar as well – don't knock it till you've tried it.

sweet potatoes

Sweet potatoes are a traditional lowland root crop in many tropical climates and were first brought to Europe by Columbus. He took them back to Spain, from whence they spread and enjoyed considerable popularity, but their appeal waned and they didn't become a common sight in Britain until the influx of immigrants from the Caribbean islands.

This created a new demand for the sweet potato, and many other delicious foods from the Caribbean, from the 1950s onwards. You'll find them today in every supermarket, street market and many corner shops. Sweet potatoes are often confused with yams, but in fact, they're a separate species; although many books describe them as alternative names for the same plant, the yam is nutritionally inferior.

Sweet potatoes are an excellent source of starch and, therefore, energy. They provide some protein, vitamin C, vitamin E and a huge amount of carotenoids, including betacarotene. It is these and the other phytochemicals in the tubers that make them such a powerful anti-cancer food. A mere 100g a day can dramatically reduce your risk of lung cancer – and this is even more important if you are a smoker or ex-smoker.

They're an extremely versatile vegetable and are wonderfully healthy for children and adults alike. A good way to introduce them to your family is to peel and cube a sweet potato and cook it together with ordinary potatoes, drain, mash with a little butter or olive oil and some grated nutmeg. They're equally delicious mashed together with parsnip or swede, and they're great just roasted in a medium oven, brushed with olive oil, and sprinkled with black pepper.

Surprisingly, they make an interesting addition to homemade juices, and combine well with other vegetables and many fruits. One of my favourite combos is apple, carrot, celery and sweet potato – which tastes better than it sounds.

tea

Nutritionally, tea contains useful quantities of vitamins E and K and small amounts of the B vitamins. It's an important source of the trace elements manganese (essential for growth, bone-building and the function of hormones and enzymes) and fluorine (essential for strong bones and teeth and protective against tooth decay). In small quantities, the astringent tannins in tea are antibacterial and help with food poisoning and other stomach infections. The tannins are also good for eye problems; a used tea bag dipped in cold water and placed over closed eyes for ten minutes gives instant relief for sticky, itchy and tired eyes.

By far the most exciting benefits of tea come from the bioflavonoids: natural plant chemicals which act as antioxidants, neutralizing the damaging free radicals that cause heart and circulatory problems. Two to four cups a day are necessary for this extra protection, and though green tea is richer in protective substances, our British brew also contains significant amounts.

When it comes to cancer prevention, green tea is certainly top of the list. Its rich content of antioxidants is only part of the cancer-prevention story, as research has revealed another amazing chemical called EGCG, a substance known to slow the growth of tumours by stopping the development of new blood vessels which would otherwise supply them with the nutrients they need to develop. There are also interesting phenolic compounds that help strengthen blood-vessel walls – which makes tea a good drink if you've got thread veins, chilblains, varicose veins or cold hands and feet.

Trouble concentrating? Have a cup of tea. Psychologists have found that something in tea (and it's not the caffeine) improves concentration and speeds up the learning process. This benefit of tea is especially marked when you're trying to concentrate on more than one job at a time. So, if you're multi-tasking, maybe a cuppa is all you need to keep your mind on the job(s).

tomatoes

The ancestral home of the tomato is the western coast region of South America, stretching from Ecuador to Peru and Chile. Even in the high mountains, wild varieties abound. and these are cherry tomatoes: the forerunners of all modern varieties.

The first domestication probably happened in Mexico, and tomatoes were introduced to Europe by the Spanish during the sixteenth century, after which they rapidly rampaged across southern Europe. As members of the *Solanaceae* family, which includes the deadly nightshade, they were treated with suspicion at first, but soon achieved their rightful place as a delicious and health-giving food.

Tomatoes are extremely rich in antioxidants, especially carotenoids such as betacarotene and lycopene, as well as vitamins C and E, making them good protectors of the cardiovascular system and against some forms of cancer. They're also extremely low in sodium and quite rich in potassium, so they are helpful in conditions such as high blood pressure and fluid retention.

There should always be a few cans of tomatoes in your cupboard, as they lose very little of their nutritional value during canning and are a great standby for instant high-nutrient sauces. A ripe tomato contains more than 200 volatile compounds that make up its unique taste and smell. Green tomatoes, however, contain a chemical called tomatine, which may trigger migraine attacks. It's also destroyed by cooking, but remains in quite high amounts in the pickled green tomatoes popular in the US.

A highly important recent discovery has been the role of lycopene, a carotenoid present in ripe tomatoes. This nutrient is known to protect men against prostate cancer – a much less common disease in Mediterranean countries where six to eight ripe tomatoes a day is the average consumption.

Interestingly, processed tomatoes contain far more lycopene than fresh ones, so tinned tomatoes, tomato sauce, ketchup and sun-dried tomatoes are extremely important, as they also protect men and women against heart disease.

turmeric

Turmeric, a member of the ginger family, is native to India and China. It's grown for its root, which is used as medicine and as the most common flavour and colour in Chinese and other Far Eastern cooking. Popular for centuries, this essential ingredient of curry powder is key to successful Asian vegetarian food – particularly lentil recipes.

Indian Ayurvedic practitioners prescribe it for eyesight, rheumatism, arthritis and also liver problems. Today's scientists are fascinated by its powerful antioxidant and protective properties, which appear to work just like the non-steroidal anti-inflammatory drugs. In addition, this spice is now thought to have powerful cancer-preventive properties, with one huge advantage: there are no side effects.

Turmeric is one spice that should be a regular part of day-to-day eating, providing substantial amounts of the highly protective and immune-boosting antioxidants and the potentially cancer-preventive effects of curcumin, one of its natural constituents.

venison

Unfortunately, childhood memories of Bambi put lots of people off this delicious and healthy meat. But venison is making a comeback. Though it's more often farmed than wild, the flavours and texture are superb when the meat is properly dressed and hung.

Nutritionally, venison contains only a third of the calories and half the fat of beef, and even less of both than chicken, so it's genuinely a healthy option. It's also an excellent source of protein, iron and B vitamins, and even when it's farmed, it is much less likely to contain antibiotics, growth hormones and many other unwanted residues.

Prime cuts should be cooked very hot and medium-rare. Otherwise, marinate before cooking in red wine, oil and herbs (common in Europe and the UK), or buttermilk.

walnuts

Walnuts are one of the most ancient of all recorded foods. Archaeologists in southwest France have found fossilized walnut shells that were roasted more than 8,000 years ago. Engraved clay tablets dating from 2,000 BC showed walnuts growing in the hanging gardens of Babylon, and both the ancient Greeks and Romans treated them as a royal food and enshrined them in their mythology.

The most widely grown variety is the English walnut, which in fact originated in Persia and got its name from the English seafarers who carried them as cargo to trade around the world. The other variety is the black walnut, native to North America but seldom grown commercially. California produces the vast majority of the world's walnuts, but these are all English walnuts introduced commercially in 1867.

Walnuts are a wonderful health-giving and nutritious snack food, providing protein, slow-release energy, potassium, magnesium, copper, zinc, and vitamins B_6 and E. But the most important constituent is the oil. They have seven times more polyunsaturated than saturated fat, and the polyunsaturates are an important source of essential fatty acids which, combined with their antioxidant properties, make them ideal for anyone with heart or circulatory disease, raised cholesterol or high blood pressure. Scientific studies in the US and Spain have found that eating a handful of walnuts a day can significantly lower cholesterol levels.

If you're lucky enough to find wet walnuts – just after harvest and before the shells have dried out – they're a real delicacy. Although just as healthy when dried, eat them either straight from the shell or chopped into cakes, biscuits, salads and other recipes.

Walnut oil is fantastic for both flavour and health-giving properties and is produced in small quantities by local growers, especially in France and Italy. There are great variations in colour and flavour and it is expensive, but a drizzle into puréed parsnips, swedes and carrots, added to bread recipes or mixed with lemon juice as a salad dressing adds a truly delicious flavour.

watercress

Hippocrates described watercress and its medicinal values in 460 BC. He even built the world's first hospital next to a stream flowing with pure spring water so that he could grow fresh watercress for his patients. The Greeks and the Romans believed watercress was a cure for madness (though taking it mixed with vinegar didn't do much for Nero). The watercress you eat today is identical in every respect to that eaten by Hippocrates, Nero and even Henry VIII.

Thanks to its high vitamin C content, it has been used since the 1500s to prevent scurvy, but there's more to this nasturtium family member. Both watercress and nasturtiums contain a benzyl mustard oil that is powerfully antibiotic but, unlike conventional antibiotics, it's kind to your friendly gut bacteria. Eating watercress and nasturtium flowers strengthens your resistance and fights chest and urinary infections.

Dr Stephen Hecht, professor of cancer prevention at the University of Minnesota, has studied the importance of watercress as a preventer of lung cancer in smokers. The best way to avoid lung cancer is to stop smoking, but those who can't should make sure that they eat a large bunch of watercress every day. These peppery-tasting leaves contain a unique chemical, phenethyl isothiocyanate, which helps neutralize the important tobacco-specific lung carcinogen NNK. This extraordinary protective chemical, also known as gluco-nasturtiin, is only released from watercress when it is chewed or chopped.

Add all this to the fact that watercress is also a useful source of iodine, which is essential for the proper functioning of the thyroid gland, and you'll understand why it isn't just a garnish on top of the steak, but a nutritious, protective and important food which should be eaten in generous quantities by everybody.

Always wash watercress thoroughly in plenty of running water to remove any residual grit or bacteria. It makes great soup, wonderful sauce to go with fish, is delicious in salads and turns a mundane sandwich into a taste sensation.

wheat

Wheat is a vitally important staple food in the Western diet. The majority of wheat ends up as flour and, finally, bread. Although bread consumption is declining, it still accounts for a quarter of all the protein in the British diet. One hundred years ago, up to three-quarters of the population's protein came from bread.

In addition to protein, wheat provides energy, B vitamins and minerals, but it doesn't contain vitamins A, C or B_{12}. For the real taste of wheat, just compare a fresh loaf made from organically grown, wholegrain flour with nothing added but a pinch of salt and fresh yeast, with the white, cotton-wool, full-of-additives variety made from refined flour that has come from the agribusiness – this flour is from wheat grown on artificially fertilized and monocropped soil and sprayed with pesticides, insecticides and fungicides.

Although refined wheat flour is fortified with some lost nutrients, zinc, magnesium, B_6, pyridoxine, vitamin E and fibre are not replaced.

People with coeliac disease cannot eat wheat as it contains gluten, and there are others who don't tolerate this cereal very well. In fact, however, few of those claiming wheat allergy actually have it; it's more likely to be an intolerance often due to over-consumption, as in recent years pasta, pizza and burgers in buns have come to dominate our eating habits.

It's a shame that we can't eat more of the same foods our ancestors did. A centuries-old British dish called frumenty was the perfect meal for millions of farm labourers in years gone by: whole wheat grains were baked overnight in the ashes of the fire (which burst open the grains) and then set into a thick jelly, which was eaten with milk, spices, honey, currants or raisins.

The wheatgerm left behind when white flour is milled is a rich source of the vitamin B complex and vitamin E, which makes it an excellent food supplement, especially for invalids and convalescents.

wine

When the French raise a glass of wine in a toast, they say *à votre santé* – 'to your health' – and those French certainly know a thing or two about the health benefits of booze. Red wine is one factor in the Mediterranean Diet that is known to protect against heart disease.

In most parts of the world as well as France, the drinker's toast is to their companion's good health – *saluté, skøl, prost, lekhayyim* – but here in the UK it's more likely to be an uninspiring 'cheers' or 'bottoms up'. That's a pity, because sensible amounts of wine are extremely beneficial and there's nothing new in that. Our most ancient ancestors discovered the art of fermentation and used their alcoholic drinks for the relief of pain. The ancient Greeks and Romans added herbs and spices to wine for medicinal purposes, and even the Bible is littered with references to the medical properties of alcohol.

French scientists have shown that men drinking moderate amounts of red wine on a regular basis have thirty percent less risk of death from all causes than heavy drinkers or total abstainers. Red grapes are an extremely rich source of natural antioxidants known as phenolic compounds, and these are known to be protective against a wide range of heart and circulatory diseases. These wines are often matured in oak casks, so they absorb even more of the natural antioxidants from the wood.

There's a good reason to enjoy Chardonnay, Sauvignon Blanc, Pinot Grigio and all the delicious white wines, too: they may be good for your lungs. Dr H Schunemann from the University of Buffalo, New York, has been studying lung function. Volunteers were questioned about their alcohol consumption, and after allowing for lifestyle, height, weight, eating habits and smoking, those drinking wine rather than other alcoholic beverages had healthier lungs. The white-wine-drinkers had the best lungs of all.

yogurt

Yogurt in some form or other has been made since time immemorial. The ancient Bedouin found that the combination of heat and movement (and, obviously, a few good bacteria) fermented the milk in their goatskin bags. The resulting yogurt then kept for days.

Most commercial yogurts start out as pasteurized milk inoculated with cultures of beneficial bacteria such as *Lactobacillus acidophilus* or *bulgaricus*, *Bifidobacteria* or *Streptococcus thermophilus*. Yet many yogurt products are then pasteurized again and contain none of the live and beneficial organisms that give yogurt its unique properties.

Live, or 'bio' yogurts contain health-giving bacteria which synthesize B vitamins, biotin, folic acid and B_{12}. They increase absorption of calcium and magnesium, and keep your bowels regular. These 'good bugs' also attack and destroy the 'bad guys' that cause food poisoning.

Because antibiotics kill all bacteria, good and bad, they should always be taken with a daily carton of live yogurt to help prevent diarrhoea. Yogurt also actively encourages the synthesis of B vitamins, thus helping to prevent the depression that commonly follows antibiotic therapy.

Yogurt is an excellent source of calcium. One 150g carton provides 210mg – well over a quarter of the minimum daily adult requirement – and for weight-conscious women, low-fat varieties contain even more, at 285mg per 150g pot. Yogurt also supplies small traces of vitamin D, which is essential for the absorption of calcium, making it an even more important source.

Veterinary scientists have found that the 'probiotics' (good bugs) present in yogurt produce enzymes that are absorbed directly through the gut wall, which strengthens the immune defences.

A daily live yogurt is a huge health bonus. Choose a plain variety and add your own fruit to avoid sugar, preservatives and other chemicals.

vitamins & minerals

It's less than a century since these essential nutrients were discovered, yet today, shelves groan under a vast array of vitamin and mineral supplements. Do you really need them? For some people, the answer is yes – and there's nothing wrong with a daily multivitamin. However, the key to good health is to get everything you need from food, which is why this section includes a selection of the most important health-enhancing nutrients we know of.

calcium

Calcium is vital for the formation and continuing strength of bones and teeth. This is of even greater importance during pregnancy, breastfeeding, childhood and for teenagers. In later life, women are at risk of osteoporosis (brittle-bone disease) caused by too little calcium in the diet and poor absorption.

Protecting bones begins in childhood, with a diet that contains calcium-rich foods. Encourage children to be active, play sport, get plenty of fresh air and sunshine; as you get older, these activities become even more important. Pregnant and nursing mothers need a good store of calcium. During your thirties, make a super effort to keep up some sort of regular exercise regime. It should be weight-bearing, to strengthen the bones, like tennis, dancing, keep-fit, walking or even energetic housework.

During menopause, women need extra calcium with vitamin D. Calcium also helps relieve the symptoms of PMS, helps prevent muscle cramp and is important as a regulator of the heart rate and blood-clotting.

A glass of milk, a carton of yogurt and 60g of cheese provide the 1,000mg of calcium you should get each day. Use low-fat versions and also eat plenty of tinned sardines (with bones), lots of greens and dried fruit, nuts, beans, and plenty of watercress and parsley. Your body needs sunlight to make vitamin D, without which it can't absorb calcium, so get outdoors and remember to eat plenty of oily fish: the best nutritional source of vitamin D.

Dairy products contain the most easily absorbed calcium, though there's virtually none in butter, double cream or cream cheese. Some vegetables, like spinach and beet greens, contain oxalic acid which prevents the absorption of calcium, and wholegrain cereals, nuts and pulses contain phytic acid, which can also interfere with calcium absorption. Sprinkling bran all over your breakfast cereals seriously reduces the calcium absorbed from the milk for the same reason. Colas and other fizzy drinks contain phosphoric acid that seriously increases the amount of calcium eliminated by the body.

Although the RDA is 800mg per day, the optimum intake should be around 1,000mg, rising to 1,200mg during pregnancy and breastfeeding. The cheapest form of calcium supplements are made from calcium carbonate, but the body can't get much of the calcium from these products. It's far more effective to pay a little more for calcium citrate, from which your body extracts twice as much of the mineral.

best sources
Cheese • Canned sardines • Tofu • Seaweed • Sesame seeds • Almonds • Figs • Yogurt • Semi-skimmed milk

folic acid

Folic acid, a member of the vitamin B group of nutrients, is found in a wide variety of foods and is best-known for its ability to prevent spina bifida in newborn babies. Unfortunately, it's the first three months of pregnancy that are crucial in the development of the baby's spine and when having adequate folic acid is so important. Many women don't realize that they are pregnant until the second or third month. In spite of the wide availability of folic acid, few people manage to get the 200 micrograms they need each day from their diet. Folic acid is also needed for the body's production of healthy red blood cells.

Latest research shows that it also plays a key role in the prevention of heart disease by controlling the amount of homocysteine in the blood. High levels of this naturally occurring chemical are known to be a factor which increases the risk of fatal heart attacks. Anaemia may be caused by getting too little folic acid and a supplement of 200 micrograms a day can soon help improve the condition and overcome the symptoms of severe tiredness.

After the menopause takes place the blood levels of homocysteine tend to increase, with a related increase in the risk of osteoporosis. For this reason it is extremely important for any women not having periods (for whatever reason) to make sure they eat a regular selection of folic-acid-rich foods. It's not advisable to take large amounts of folic acid – more than 500 micrograms daily – for long periods without discussing this with your GP, as at this level it may mask the symptoms of pernicious anaemia. Folic acid can also interfere with medicine taken for epilepsy, so epileptics must also talk to their doctor before taking it.

It's always best to take folic acid supplements together with food as this improves absorption. Alcohol, the pill, aspirin, anti-inflammatory drugs and medicines for non-insulin dependent diabetes can all interfere with the absorption of folic acid.

best sources
Liver (but not to be eaten in pregnancy) • Fortified cereals • Beetroot • Brussels sprouts • Peanuts (fresh, unsalted) • Garbanzo (black-eyed) beans • Spinach

iron

Iron is one of the most important of all nutrients; without it, your body can't make haemoglobin, the substance that gives blood its red colour. It's haemoglobin that transports oxygen via the blood to every living cell in the body. As well as circulating in the blood, iron is also stored in the liver and other organs, and is available to make up for day-to-day variations in the amount of iron in the diet. Unfortunately, most women of child-bearing age and forty percent of schoolchildren do not get enough iron from their food and are consequently likely to become anaemic, one of the commonest nutritional disorders.

The iron RDA is 14mg, but this is set at around ten times the actual amount you need, because iron is poorly absorbed from most foods. Women need twice as much as men to compensate for their monthly blood loss, and they need even more during pregnancy to make sure that enough is passed to the baby and stored by the mother in preparation for breastfeeding.

Iron from animal sources is better absorbed than that from all other foodstuffs, and all iron is better absorbed in the presence of vitamin C. A glass of fresh orange juice with breakfast and plenty of fresh fruits, vegetables and salads spread throughout the day can make a substantial difference to the levels of iron in the blood.

A number of factors make it even more difficult for your body to extract iron from food. Tannins from tea are an important factor, especially in older people whose diets may be poor and who tend to drink large amounts of strong tea. Wholegrain cereals, peas, beans and cocoa contain plenty of iron, but this is poorly absorbed because they also have high levels of phytates, which reduce absorption. Bran and high-bran cereals act in the same way. Although spinach is a very rich source of iron, you'd have to eat a kilo to get as much of the mineral as you would from 100g of beef. Excessive fatigue, hair loss, pale skin and gums, feeling tired, headaches and shortness of breath are all signs of iron deficiency.

Natural supplements such as ferrous gluconate are less likely to cause digestive problems. One of my favourites is Spatone Iron (plus), a naturally occurring Welsh mineral water with a well-absorbed iron content. Conveniently packed in 20ml sachets, each one provide your daily need of absorbed iron. Do not exceed 15mg per day without professional advice. If you think you may be anaemic, see your GP to establish the underlying cause.

best sources
Seaweed • Pheasant • Lambs liver • Beef • Sardines • Mussels • Brazil nuts • Balti vegetable curry

potassium

Of all essential minerals, potassium is probably the least understood by the general public, but it is absolutely essential for many reasons. It is needed to maintain the balance between acids and alkalis in all body fluids and cells – a balance that is vital for survival. Potassium also plays a key role in the transmission of nerve impulses throughout the body, and in the prevention of calcium being lost in the urine. The other major function of this mineral is to promote muscle activity and prevent cramp, and it's in this area that most people will have heard about its importance.

Athletes have always been plagued by cramp. Until recently, the common perception was that cramp was caused by the amount of salt lost through sweating. Yet not only is salt ineffective in the relief or prevention of cramp, but it also increases the risk of high blood pressure, strokes and heart disease. Moreover, excessive salt intake causes oedema: the swelling of the hands, feet and legs due to fluid retention.

We're now used to seeing tennis players munching on bananas in the middle of a match, and footballers and other professional athletes packing them in their sports kits. This is because bananas supply easily digestible carbohydrates for energy and loads of potassium to prevent cramp and keep their muscles working efficiently.

Excessive consumption of sodium in any form, taking water tablets (diuretics), cortisone medication and too much alcohol can all reduce potassium levels. All fruits and vegetables, as well as instant coffee and red wine, contain potassium. But boiling your vegetables halves the content, as the mineral ends up in the cooking water, so make sure you use it in soups and gravies.

Blood loss, chronic diarrhoea or vomiting, diabetes, kidney disease or prolonged use of laxatives or diuretics can all cause potassium deficiency. This can be a particular worry in older people who tend to have a lower nutrient intake. Lack of potassium can cause muscle weakness, cramp, disorientation, mental confusion, depression and, if severe, heart attacks. Potassium supplements can help lower high blood pressure and reduce the risk of strokes, irregular heart rhythms and heart attacks.

The average adult needs 3,500mg of potassium daily. Supplements of 2,000mg to 3,000mg per day are adequate for the majority of people.

best sources
Bananas • Dried apricots • Baked jacket potato • Prunes • Almonds • Dry-roasted peanuts • Stir-fry vegetables (courgette, Chinese cabbage, leeks, onion, garlic, spinach) • Tomato purée • Grilled chicken breast

selenium

Selenium is a trace mineral, which means the body only needs tiny amounts each day, but a lack of it can be catastrophic. There's no official recommended daily amount, but most experts agree that 70 micrograms is the minimum we require. Worryingly, the average Brit today only gets around 30 micrograms, and this has serious implications.

Selenium is one of the major protective antioxidants that helps prevent damage to individual body cells. It's vital for the prevention of heart disease, and selenium deficiency is a major factor in the development of prostate cancer in men. Cancers of the lung and bowel are also thought to be associated with low intakes of selenium. Selenium is part of body's general defence mechanism, but it's also involved in the function of natural enzymes that regulate many of our bodily functions, including blood clotting and the protection of DNA – the genetic blueprint of every cell.

The amount of selenium that ends up in the food you eat depends firstly on how much there was in the soil in which the foods were grown or on which animals grazed, and secondly on the amount of processing to which the food has been subjected. Traditionally in the UK, most of our selenium was found in bread made from Canadian and North American wheat; the soil's selenium ended up in our bread. Now, thanks to the EU, our flour is made from European wheat with much lower selenium levels. What's more, our diets have become more and more reliant on processed and, therefore, deficient foods.

Virtually everyone in the UK needs to increase their intake of this vital mineral – particularly smokers; any man with prostate problems, poor fertility or a history of prostate cancer in the family; anyone with a family history of heart disease or any form of cancer; people with very poor diets; and vegans or vegetarians who don't pay attention to their nutrition. Selenium is also protective against many toxic chemicals as it combines with them and aids their removal from the body, so jobs that involve working with chemicals mean you need a higher intake.

Organically produced food has higher levels of selenium, and supplements are widely available in chemists and health-food stores. The mineral is best absorbed in the presence of vitamins A, C and E, but do not exceed a daily dose of 200 micrograms. It's present in most multivitamin and mineral pills.

best sources
Brazil nuts • Wholemeal bread • Oily fish • Tuna, canned in oil
• Sunflower seeds • Cooked mushrooms • Steak & kidney pie • Shrimp
• Mixed nuts & raisins

vitamin A

Vitamin A is essential for many different functions, including night vision and colour perception. It plays an important part in maintaining the body's natural defences by boosting immunity and resistance to viruses and bacteria. Another key function is the protection of mucous membranes – the linings of the mouth, nose, throat and lungs; without this vitamin, these tissues dry out and cannot perform their vital functions. Few people realize that vitamin A plays a key role in growth and bone development. It is required by men and women for fertility and reproduction. There is some evidence of its role in supporting the mechanisms of both taste and balance. Finally, vitamin A plays a key role in the growth and maintenance of healthy skin which keeps its elasticity; thus, as a bonus, it slows the development of wrinkles.

Because vitamin A is fat-soluble, the main sources are foods also containing some fats and oils. For this reason, it's essential to include fats, oils and the good food sources in the diet to make sure you get enough of this nutrient and that the body is able to absorb it. Anti-cholesterol drugs, antacids, indigestion remedies and zinc deficiency can also reduce levels of vitamin A.

The body gets its supplies of vitamin A directly from foods containing it and indirectly through the conversion of betacarotene. Betacarotene is the brightly coloured yellow pigment found in foods such as carrots, apricots, sweet potatoes and most dark- green leafy vegetables, especially spinach.

The amount of vitamin A required each day is 800 micrograms. Although liver, oily fish, butter, cheese, carrots, vegetables and even milk offer substantial amounts, many people fail to get the minimum RDA, putting their health at risk. This is especially true of young women following extreme weight-loss diets.

The body stores surplus amounts of vitamin A in fatty tissues like the liver, so excessive doses can be extremely toxic. Never exceed the recommended dose of pills containing vitamin A and don't eat extremely rich sources such as liver more than a couple of times a week. Pregnant women should avoid vitamin A supplements and liver completely. Headaches, nausea, peeling itchy skin, hair loss and bone deformities can result from overdosing.

Cancer prevention is one of the major roles of vitamin A, but it's useful for people with chronic respiratory illness such as asthma and bronchitis.

best sources
Liver • Carrots • Spinach • Butter • Eggs • Cheddar cheese
• Dried apricots • Sweet potatoes

vitamin B$_6$ (pyridoxine)

You need just 2mg of B$_6$ per day, but in spite of this nutrient being found in a large range of foods, it's quite common for people, especially women, to get less than the RDA in their diet. More importantly, larger intakes than the RDA can result in the reduction, prevention and even cure of a number of health problems. B$_6$ is essential for many chemical reactions that enable the body to use proteins and amino acids. It has a role in normal brain function, is important for red blood cells and the correct balance of the body's chemical make-up. B$_6$ is also a part of the body's system responsible for the excretion of water and the mechanism that produces energy from food. It protects against some types of anaemia and helps in stress control.

The best-known function of B$_6$ is the relief of PMS, thanks to its effect on hormone balance. It eases fluid retention, prevents mood swings, can dramatically improve depression and reduces episodes of aggressive behaviour in the days leading up to a period. Another condition that responds well to B$_6$ therapy is carpal tunnel syndrome. This type of RSI problem affects the nerves of the hand as they pass through the tissues of the wrist and can cause severe pain, burning, tingling and loss of sensation of the fingers.

Research has shown that many people who suffer chronic depression have low circulating levels of vitamin B$_6$ in their blood. My colleagues and I would certainly advise it for anyone with long-term depression. The whole of the central and peripheral nervous system needs adequate supplies of B vitamins; this group of nutrients is also helpful for the relief of chronic fatigue and Tired all the Time syndrome. In these instances, a B-complex tablet that includes B$_6$ is an invaluable part of holistic treatment.

Vitamin B$_6$ is excreted the same day you get it, so it's essential to have regular intakes. Anyone on high-protein diets, vegans, vegetarians, the elderly, women taking the pill or HRT, alcoholics and people with very low calorie intakes for any reason, need a B$_6$ supplement. This is also the case if you're taking penicillin, immunosuppressants or if you smoke.

Excessive amounts of B$_6$ can cause neurological problems, including numbness of the hands and feet, clumsiness and general inflammation of the nerves; if this happens, stop taking the supplement immediately. These side effects have been reported at doses as low as 50mg a day, but in general, the safe upper limit is 250mg daily. I recommend starting at a dose of 50-100mg daily.

best sources
Calves liver • Grilled herring • Turkey • Wheatgerm • Bananas
• Wholemeal bread • Fresh unsalted peanuts

vitamin B_{12}

B_{12} is part of the vitamin B complex which is essential for the prevention of pernicious anaemia. The RDA is only 1 microgram, which is easy to obtain from meat, fish, poultry, eggs, cheese and all animal-based foods. It is absent from virtually all plant foods except yeast extracts and fermented soy products, although it is often added to fortified breakfast cereals. For this reason, vegetarians and especially vegans should always take a daily supplement.

In order for the body to utilize B_{12}, a substance called the 'intrinsic factor', produced by the lining of the stomach, is essential, and the failure to produce enough is a common cause of pernicious anaemia. This condition used to be fatal, but it was first treated successfully with injections of liquidized raw liver – the richest source of B_{12}. In modern medicine, B_{12} itself can now be injected.

This vitamin is also needed for the production of a fatty substance called myelin, which forms a protective sheath covering all the nerves in the body. Deficiency of B_{12} reduces the amount of myelin, and as this is needed for the rapid transmission of nerve impulses, it can also result in serious neurological problems. Another function of this nutrient is the production of special enzymes which work together with folic acid. This means that vitamin B_{12} is also an essential requirement for the normal growth of babies during pregnancy and breastfeeding.

Enough vitamin B_{12} is stored in your liver to last around two years, but unless you continually replace what you're using, the reserve runs out, your bone marrow doesn't make enough healthy blood cells and the consequence is anaemia. Chronic fatigue, pale skin (especially inside the eyelids), loss of concentration, short-term memory, mood swings, sore tongue, loss of appetite, nausea, breathlessness and general weakness of arm and leg muscles can all be signs of B_{12} deficiency. Although the RDA is only 1 microgram, it's sensible to aim for 2 micrograms for children under 12, 3 micrograms for over-12s, and 5 micrograms for adults. As B_{12} is best absorbed in the presence of other vitamins, it's more effective as part of a multivitamin and mineral supplement than taken singly, unless prescribed by your health practitioner. The contraceptive pill, sleeping pills, some anti-diabetic drugs and excessive amounts of alcohol can all reduce absorption.

best sources
Liver • Duck • Roast beef sandwich • Grilled plaice • Scrambled eggs • Vegetarian Cheddar • Soya cheese • Marmite

vitamin C

Vitamin C is probably the best-known of all vitamins. Though it's by far the easiest to get in your diet, most people barely get enough each day. Vitamin C is a water-soluble vitamin found in virtually every variety of fruit and vegetable, although it is commonly linked with citrus fruits. It is a powerful antioxidant that protects every cell from damage caused by the free radicals that are by-products of pollution and natural chemical processes. A key benefit of this vitamin is the way in which it increases natural resistance to infection.

The RDA is 60mg, and while this is enough to prevent scurvy, none of the real nutrition experts believe it's anywhere near enough to promote the best-possible health. You'll get your daily allowance from a glass of orange juice, a kiwi fruit or 85g (3oz, of strawberries. For serious protection against flu, coughs and colds (an essential for smokers), avoiding cataract problems, fighting off cold sores, and to stimulate wound-healing after accidents or surgery, you need a minimum of 250mg daily – ideally 1,000mg or more.

Blackcurrants, papaya, green peppers and all green leafy vegetables are excellent sources, but for most people, a daily supplement could be the cheapest and best health insurance. Many studies have shown that vitamin C protects against infections.

The body cannot store large amounts of vitamin C, so you really need it on a daily basis. Professor Gladys Block, one of the world's leading experts on health and nutrition, says she aims for a minimum of 250mg each day, but for therapeutic purposes, for smokers, athletes, anyone in their 60s or routinely taking soluble aspirin to protect their heart, 500mg to 1,000mg is the optimum level. It's also important for women on the pill and anyone on long-term antibiotics or steroid drugs to increase their vitamin C intake, both from food and supplements.

Vitamin C is best absorbed when eaten with good sources of bioflavonoids. Bioflavaonoids are a large group of naturally occurring chemicals found in many fruits and vegetables. In citrus fruits, for example, they are present in the pith between the skin and the flesh. The highest concentrations are in the most brightly coloured produce. Bioflavonoids improve the body's absorption of vitamin C, and this is helped even more if you eat foods containing calcium and magnesium.

best sources
Strawberries • Papaya • Kiwi fruit • Green peppers (raw) • Oranges • Broccoli (cooked) • Blackcurrants (cooked) • Coleslaw (homemade)

vitamin D

Vitamin D is the vital key to strong, healthy bones. Together with sufficient calcium, it's essential for your bones as, without it, the body cannot absorb calcium from food. In childhood, a lack of vitamin D prevents bones from hardening and causes rickets, a condition that leads to bone deformity, bow legs and disability. A lack of vitamin D in adults results in osteomalacia: softening of the bones. It doesn't matter how much calcium you get from your diet or supplements; without vitamin D, the end result will almost certainly be osteoporosis, causing loss of height and a greatly increased risk of fractures of the hip, spine and almost any other bone in your body.

The body can manufacture its own vitamin D and this takes place when skin is exposed to ultraviolet light from the sun. Vitamin D formed in this way is stored in the skin and slowly released into the blood, then converted into a hormone-like chemical in the liver and kidneys. It's this active form of vitamin D that the body needs to extract calcium from food. If you don't get enough sunshine on your skin – ten to fifteen minutes a day on arms, legs, and face without sun block; early morning or late afternoon is perfectly safe – and you're not eating sufficient of the vitamin D-rich foods, then you can't maintain strong bones or teeth.

Those at special risk are the elderly, vegetarians, vegans, breastfeeding and pregnant women, and anyone who spends little time outdoors during the summer. The Asian community is often at risk due to traditional clothing, diet and lifestyle. Anybody in these groups or with a family history or diagnosis of osteoporosis must take a vitamin D supplement. But be careful: vitamin D at ten times the daily need can be toxic to children; twenty-five times is dangerous for adults. Don't give more than a teaspoon of cod liver oil to the kids each day or exceed this amount during pregnancy. The official RDA is 5 micrograms but 10 micrograms daily is a much more sensible target to aim for, especially if you're over sixty and your diet is not a good source of vitamin D.

Few foods contain vitamin D, but this fat-soluble nutrient is abundant in oily fish. There are modest amounts in eggs and it is added to margarines. There is no vitamin D in any fruit, vegetables and other plant foods. Ten micrograms will be obtained from 1 teaspoon of cod liver oil, 45g of herring or kipper, 55g mackerel, 80g canned salmon or tuna or 135g canned sardines.

best sources
Cod liver oil • Herring & kippers • Smoked mackerel • Sardines: grilled & canned • Grilled trout • Grilled salmon steak • Eggs

vitamin E

Even though this fat-soluble vitamin is found in a wide selection of foods, many people do not get the RDA of 10mg from their normal diets. Generally, the body builds up its own stores of fat-soluble vitamins, but vitamin E is an exception – which is why it's so important to get adequate amounts on a regular basis.

Vitamin E is one of the most powerful of natural antioxidants and is essential for protecting the body from the damage done by free radicals. It's especially important for cell walls, skin, muscles, nerves, blood vessels and the heart. This vitamin is also believed to be important for fertility, and high doses have been shown to increase the number of sperm in men with low sperm counts. High doses of vitamin E (more than 200mg) should not be taken by anyone with high blood pressure or heart disease without advice from their GP.

Taking the pill, environmental pollution and the action of the unhealthy trans-fats in many margarines can all interfere with vitamin E levels. Cholesterol-lowering drugs and excessive intake of iron or copper can also lower the body's levels of vitamin E. For this reason, vitamin E supplements should be taken at least four hours apart from mineral supplements that include iron and copper.

The body's absorption of vitamin E is increased by vitamin C and the mineral selenium. Interestingly, many of the nuts and seeds rich in vitamin E are also good sources of selenium. Eating vitamin C-rich foods at the same time as those containing vitamin E helps ensure maximum absorption.

Vitamin E is protective against heart disease, some forms of cancer (especially of the lung) and, together with vitamin C, may be useful in the treatment of cataracts. Some long-term vitamin E studies have shown that the heart-protective benefits are better when high intakes of vitamin E come from food rather than just relying on supplements. This is probably because foods rich in vitamin E also tend to be those with high levels of other naturally protective antioxidants.

Loss of libido, low levels of stamina, varicose veins, piles, thread veins, repeated infections and slow wound-healing may all indicate a shortage of this essential vitamin.

best sources
Wheatgerm oil • Avocado • Baked sweet potato • Wheatgerm • Sunflower seeds • Rape-seed oil • Hazelnuts • Blackberries • Tomato purée

zinc

Zinc is a greatly ignored trace element that is essential for children's growth, wound-healing, healthy sex organs, reproduction, insulin production and natural resistance to disease. Zinc is also essential for the senses of taste and smell and it plays a role in the creation of a good appetite. Without adequate zinc, men are not able to produce sufficient sperm and may become infertile.

One of the best-known folklore aphrodisiacs is the oyster, and although most people scoff at the thought of any foods being actual aphrodisiacs, oysters are the richest of all sources of zinc. Casanova reputedly ate up to seventy a day, usually enjoying them in the bath with his latest conquest.

Brittle nails, especially with white flecks, are nearly always attributed to a lack of calcium. In fact, there's very little calcium in nails and the most common cause is a lack of zinc. Meat, shellfish, fish, cheese and eggs are all good sources, but although wholemeal bread, nuts, wholegrains and some vegetables contain reasonable amounts of zinc, it is difficult for the body to extract much of it, due to their content of other chemicals such as phytates and oxalic acid.

Taking the pill and long-term use of the antibiotic tetracycline, often prescribed for acne, also reduce absorption of this mineral. Vegetarians and vegans may be seriously short of zinc, and this is a worry as there are no readily available stores in the body which can make up for fluctuations in your daily consumption. This can be an important factor for children and nursing mothers, as they both need extra supplies – children for growth and repair of damaged cells and mums for the high content in their milk.

Acne, PMS, post-natal depression, loss of appetite, slow wound-healing, poor hair and nails, anorexia nervosa, slow growth in children, hyperactivity and loss of the sense of smell are all signs that extra zinc may be needed. Prostate health in men is highly dependent on adequate supplies of zinc, and a deficiency can lead to enlargement of the prostate and, especially when combined with selenium deficiency, a greater risk of prostate cancer. The RDA is 15mg per day.

best sources
Oysters • Calves liver • Sardines • Roast beef • Pumpkin seeds • Crab • Eggs • Cheese

vitamins and modern living

Healthy eating means consuming plenty of essential nutrients. However, most people in the UK currently don't get enough, as shown by the following statistics.

- Over ninety-five percent of adults are deficient in folic acid
- Sixty percent of women are short of iron
- Ninety percent of men and women miss out on vitamin B_6
- Fifty percent of women are short of vitamin A
- Fifty percent of children don't get enough of vitamins A, B_{12}, D, E or folic acid
- Many adults and children are short of calcium, iron, zinc and selenium
- Twenty percent of four- to eighteen-year-olds eat no fruit

risks of the typical british diet

- High blood pressure, strokes and circulatory disease
- Gallstones, digestive problems and bowel cancer
- Arthritis, back pain and osteoporosis
- Hormone-linked problems such as acne, painful periods, low sperm counts and reduced fertility

superfeasts

super celery juice

Vitality means a strong heart and boundless energy. That's what you get from this wonderful juice: instant energy from the natural sugars in the pears, which also supply special fibre to lower cholesterol and protect the heart; slow-release energy and piles of protein from the almonds; and a subtle, bitter-sweet flavour to revitalize the palate.

2 firm Conference pears
2 celery sticks, with leaves
115g or 4oz fresh young spinach leaves
1 tablespoon ground almonds

1 Juice the fresh ingredients.
2 Stir in the ground almonds.
3 Adjust the consistency if necessary by adding mineral water.
4 Serve decorated with mint leaves.

RICH IN Soluble fibre from the pears, diuretic properties from the celery, cancer-protecting agents from the spinach, protein from the almonds

auntie leiki's sorrel soup

serves
4–6

My Auntie Leiki was a soup supremo, and this was one of her favourites, made from a simple herb she grew in the garden. It grows like a weed, survives through the winter and has a wonderfully fresh flavour, almost like grass. This was her recipe for anyone needing a vitality boost, convalescing or just feeling below par. It provides a huge boost to the immune system from onions and leeks, vital iron from the sorrel, and masses of minerals from homemade vegetable stock.

2 medium onions, chopped
3 medium leeks, finely sliced
4 tablespoons rape-seed (Canola) oil
450g or 1lb peeled and diced potato
1.2 litres or 2 pints homemade vegetable stock
2 large bunches of sorrel (or rocket), cleaned and finely chopped
300ml or 10fl oz crème fraîche or single cream

1 Simmer the potatoes in the stock until tender.
2 In a separate pan, sweat the onions and leeks gently in oil.
3 Pour the onion mixture into the potatoes and stock. Add the sorrel, keeping 2 tablespoons for garnish. Remove from heat and allow to infuse for 15 minutes.
4 Liquidize in a processor or with a mouli.
5 Return to one pan. Add the crème fraîche or cream and stir well.
6 Reheat to serve hot, but do *not* boil. Alternatively, chill and serve cold.
7 Sprinkle with finely chopped sorrel leaves.

RICH IN Iron from the sorrel, an excellent balance of omega-3 and omega-6 fatty acids from the rape-seed oil, immune-boosting chemicals from the onions and leeks, and calcium from the crème fraîche or cream

spicy veggie stew

I'm not a vegetarian; give me a bacon buttie any Sunday morning. But I do like vegetarian meals and probably don't eat meat more than two or three times a week. This is a particular favourite – something I thought up just because we had some leftovers and store-cupboard staples sitting there waiting to be cooked.

1 medium onion

4 tablespoons olive oil

1 teaspoon each cumin and garam masala

½ teaspoon cinnamon

1 small squash, such as butternut, or a chunk of pumpkin, peeled, deseeded and diced

1 small sweet potato, peeled and diced

225g or 8oz can chopped tomatoes

300ml or 10fl oz homemade stock

200g or 7oz baby leaf spinach

115g or 4oz Camargue rice

1 Start to cook rice as per instructions. Camargue takes about 30 minutes.

2 Sweat the onion in the oil. Add the cumin and cinnamon and cook for 2 minutes.

3 Soften the squash and potato gently in the onion mixture for 4 to 5 minutes.

4 Pour on the stock and tomatoes. Simmer until nearly tender.

5 Stir in the garam masala, pile on the spinach and simmer, covered, for 3 minutes, or until leaves wilt into a green covering.

6 Serve the vegetables on the rice.

RICH IN Heart-protective lycopene from the tomatoes, vitality-boosting spices, folic acid and protective carotenoids from the spinach, betacarotene from the sweet potato

curried fish with rice & peas

Yah man! Rice and peas is a traditional favourite among West Indians – and quite rightly so. It's usually made with black-eye beans, but here I've made it with green peas. It's still a wonderful combination of favours. I've also added fish and curry powder to make it a sort of kedgeree. You'll love it.

1 small onion, sliced
1 garlic clove
3 tablespoons olive oil
115g or 4oz each cod and haddock fillet, cut into chunks
2 teaspoons curry powder
400ml or 14fl oz stock mixed with 150ml or 5fl oz coconut milk
115g or 4oz rice
200g or 7oz frozen peas

1 Sweat the onion and garlic in the oil.
2 Sprinkle in the curry powder, add 2 tablespoons of the stock and mix thoroughly.
3 Add the rice and rest of the stock and simmer until the liquid is almost absorbed: about 15 to 20 minutes.
4 Mix in the fish and peas and cook until everything is tender: about five minutes.

RICH IN Energy from the rice and peas, minerals and protein from the fish, vitality-boosting and protective spices from the curry

smoked fish pasta

It may sound strange to put this amount of smoked fish into a pasta meal, but believe me, it tastes wonderful – particularly with the complementary tartness of the grapefruit and the fresh crunchiness of the green beans.

175g or 6oz organic penne
1 medium courgette, finely sliced
115g or 4oz French beans, finely snipped
1 grapefruit, segmented, plus 100ml or 3½fl oz fresh grapefruit juice
3 tablespoons extra-virgin olive oil
280g or 10oz smoked mackerel
55g or 2oz smoked salmon
4 tablespoons mixed flat-leaf parsley and chives, finely chopped and snipped

1 Cook the pasta according to the packet instructions.
2 Simmer the courgettes and beans until just tender.
3 Mix the oil and grapefruit juice. Stir it into the pasta and cool.
4 Flake the mackerel. Chop the smoked salmon.
5 Combine all ingredients. Season to taste, and sprinkle with the herbs.

RICH IN Energy, protein and bone-protecting vitamin D from the fish, slow-release carbohydrates from the pasta, vitamin C from the beans and grapefruit, heart-protective properties from the extra-virgin olive oil

prune & cranberry duck

serves
4

This unusual way of cooking duck is extremely simple, and you'll find prepared duck breasts in most supermarkets. It's a perfect dish if you're entertaining, as you can prepare it in advance and reheat it when you're ready. It provides excellent protein and is massively protective against heart disease and cancer, thanks to the prunes and cranberries.

115g or 4oz dried cranberries
4 tablespoons olive oil
2 large Spanish onions, finely diced
2 tablespoons wholemeal flour
4 duck breasts
2 large sprigs fresh thyme
200ml or 7fl oz orange juice
150ml or 5fl oz dry white wine
85g or 3oz ready-to-eat prunes

1 Pour enough boiling water over the cranberries just to cover them. Leave in a bowl.
2 Heat 2 tablespoons of the oil in a large frying pan.
3 Sauté the onions gently for 5 minutes.
4 Add the flour and cook gently, stirring continuously, for another 2 minutes.
5 Trim any fat off the duck breasts and flatten slightly with the back of a wooden spoon.
6 Heat the rest of the oil in another pan. Sauté the duck breasts, two at a time, for 5 minutes on each side. Set aside and reserve.

7 Drain the cranberries, reserving the liquid.

8 Strip the leaves off the thyme and chop finely.

9 Over a gentle heat, gradually pour the orange juice, wine and cranberry liquid into the onion and flour mixture.

10 Add the thyme and duck breasts.

11 Snip the prunes into cranberry-size pieces and add to the pan.

12 Cover and simmer for about 30 minutes, until duck is tender.

RICH IN Cancer-fighting agents in the cranberries and prunes, protein from the duck, antioxidants from the onions, vitamin C from the orange juice, cleansing properties from the thyme

nutty about chicken

It was 1964 and I was in southern Portugal. I stopped for lunch in a small local café and they produced this big bowl of chicken with pine kernels. I thought they were nuts to combine these two ingredients, but I loved it. I hope you will, too.

4 organic on-the-bone chicken thighs, skins removed

3 tablespoons peanut oil

1 large sweet onion, finely chopped

2 garlic cloves, finely chopped

1 slice of organic stone-ground bread, crusts removed, cubed

1 teaspoon allspice mixed with 8 crushed peppercorns

55g or 2oz pine nuts

200ml or 7fl oz dry red wine

1 Brown the chicken in hot oil. Remove and set aside.

2 Turn down the heat and soften the onion and garlic in the remaining oil.

3 Add the bread cubes and fry at a higher heat until golden.

4 Mix in the spices and pine nuts and fry for 1 minute, stirring constantly. Then add the wine.

5 Put the chicken pieces in a casserole. Add the wine mixture and cook at 200°C or 400°F or gas mark 6 for 40 minutes, adding more wine or water if necessary.

RICH IN Easily absorbed iron and zinc from the chicken, antioxidants from the red wine (but don't have more than two glasses a day), antibacterials from the onions, vitalizing properties from the allspice and peppercorns

fig fantasy

Fresh figs are the ultimate succulent, sensuous, delicious and vitality-boosting fruit. They're full of nutrients and also have a natural sugar content, which provides an instant boost. They may seem expensive when you see them in the supermarket, but look in any street market and they'll be much better value. In any case, this quick and simple dish is well worth any extra expense.

6 ripe figs (or as many as you can find because you're bound to want more)
4 tablespoons of brandy
225g or 8oz soft goat cheese, a cylindrical variety cut into 12 x 5mm or
   ¼-inch slices.

1 Slice the figs lengthwise. Arrange them in a heatproof dish so that
   they fit snugly.
2 Spoon the brandy equally onto each fruit.
3 Top each fig half with a slice of goat cheese.
4 Put under preheated hot grill for 5 minutes.

RICH IN Betacarotene, iron and potassium from the figs, calcium in the goat cheese, circulation-boosting properties in the brandy

a parcel of salmon

So simple. Salmon is very inexpensive these days, and this is the quickest way to cook it. It comes out of the oven sweet and succulent and goes really well with mashed potato and a simple salad such as cucumber and capers or lettuce with avocado.

4 salmon fillets
55g or 2oz unsalted butter, cubed
4 small spring onions, cleaned and cut diagonally
1 regular glass of white wine
Juice of 1 lemon
4 fennel fronds

1 Wash the salmon fillets and dry on kitchen paper.
2 Cut four pieces of kitchen foil large enough to make generous parcels around the fish.
3 Put the fish into the foil.
4 Divide the butter, spring onions, wine, lemon juice and fennel among the parcels.
5 Close the foil into loose, airtight parcels and put into the oven at 180°C or 350°F or gas mark 4 for 20 minutes.

RICH IN Protein and a balanced mixture of omega-3 and omega-6 fatty acids from the salmon, essential trace minerals from the fennel, antioxidants from the spring onion, vitamin C from the lemon

beer stew

This wonderfully warming stew is the epitome of comfort food, but it's fantastic vitality food, too, thanks to all the goodness in the energy-giving ingredients.

450g or 1lb lean organic stewing beef, cubed
4 tablespoons plain flour, seasoned with pepper
2 garlic cloves, finely chopped
1 medium onion, finely chopped
3 tablespoons olive oil
300ml or ½ pint Guinness, or other dark ale
450g or 1lb mixed root vegetables, peeled and diced
1 bouquet garni
1 tablespoon chopped sage leaves

1 Toss the meat in the seasoned flour.
2 Put the garlic and onion into a large frying pan with the olive oil and sauté gently until soft.
3 Add the beef and fry gently until browned all over.
4 Pour in the ale and tip in the vegetables. Add water if the mixture isn't covered.
5 Add the bouquet garni.
6 Cover and simmer until the meat is tender, about 2 hours, topping up with more ale or water if it seems to be drying out.
7 Add the sage leaves just before taking it off the heat.

RICH IN Conjugated linoleic acid, a powerful cancer-fighting fat only present in organically reared beef; fibre, potassium, folic acid and vitamins from the root vegetables, particularly parsnips; silicon, from the beer, known to protect against osteoporosis; phytoestrogens from the sage, to regulate menstrual and menopausal problems

lamb, lentil & carrot casserole

It always surprises me how people shun cheaper cuts of meat. Shank of lamb is so delicious because so much of the meat is near the bone – and it is amazingly good value. It's also rich in protein and B vitamins and is an excellent food for those with anaemia. Here, it's cooked with those wonderful Puy lentils: little sparks of energy which contain iron, zinc and calcium, made more easily absorbed by the vitamin C in the carrots.

3 tablespoons olive oil
2–3 lamb shanks, about 1.6kg or 3½lbs in weight
1 onion, finely chopped
2 garlic cloves, finely chopped
3 carrots, sliced
700ml or 1¼pints vegetable or meat stock
2 bay leaves
1 bouquet garni
275g or 9½oz Puy lentils

1 Heat the oil in a large, ovenproof casserole, add the lamb and brown all over.
2 Remove and set aside.
3 Put the onion, garlic and carrots into the casserole and cook gently for 5 minutes.
4 Return the lamb to the casserole, pour in the stock, add the bay leaves, bouquet garni and Puy lentils.
5 Cover and cook for 2 hours at 200°C or 400°F or gas mark 6, adding more stock or water if it starts to dry out.
6 To serve, arrange the lamb on top of the lentils and vegetables on a large platter. Everyone can then pull the meat off the bone and help themselves to the delicious vegetable sauce.

RICH IN Protein and iron from the lamb, slow-release energy, fibre and phytoestrogens from the lentils, betacarotene from the carrots

peanut butter pick-me-up

This smoothie is a real get-you-up-and-go drink. Use it as a brilliant start to the day, a pick-me-up when you get home in the evening or a real vitality boost when your spirits are flagging at lunchtime. Kids will love this, too.

6 apples, washed, uncored and quartered

2 bananas, peeled

2 tablespoons peanut butter

2 mint leaves, finely chopped

1 Put the first three ingredients into a blender and whizz until smooth.

2 Serve with the mint leaves scattered on top.

RICH IN The soluble fibre pectin from the apples, slow-release carbohydrates in the bananas, protein, iron, folic acid, vitamin E and magnesium from the peanut butter, digestive properties from the mint

quick vitality drinks

Drinks are a great aid in the battle for vitality and feeling well. As everyone knows, the great British cuppa seems to be the answer to every emotion; in times of happiness we celebrate with tea, in times of stress we make a stronger brew, in times of difficulty we just add a few spoons of sugar. Whether you're dealing with triumph or disaster, out comes the teapot.

While it's true that tea contains modest amounts of caffeine, lots of tannins and some important minerals, there are lots of natural alternatives which, in drink form, have an extremely rapid effect on your emotional state. For instant vitality, especially during the winter months, ginger tea is a great energy booster. The best way to make it is to peel and grate half an inch of fresh ginger, add boiling water, cover and let stand for ten minutes, strain and sip slowly. If you find it a bit too strong for your palate, add a teaspoon of maple syrup or honey. Ginger has an instant stimulating effect on the blood circulation and you'll feel the difference within minutes of taking this delicious drink. As a bonus this is also a great cure for travel sickness, early morning sickness in pregnancy and for the nausea following an anaesthetic.

For really interesting drinks it's worth investing in a juicer and you can buy excellent ones like Kenwood, Phillips or Moulinex for around £40. If you want a real pick-me-up, for instance, add three teaspoons of guarana extract to the juice of a mango, a pawpaw, half a pineapple and two kiwi fruit. This provides a mountainous supply of vitamin C, together with masses of stimulating enzymes from the tropical fruits.

vitality feasts

mad about pasta

It's true, you do use more energy eating celery than you get from it, but there's a hidden benefit. The natural chemicals it contains are cleansing and revitalizing. Followed by energy-giving pasta, brain-boosting essential fatty acids from the fish and healing enzymes from the pineapple, this a gold-star vitality feast.

- Super Celery Juice, *see* page 125
- Smoked Fish Pasta, *see* page 129
- Fresh pineapple topped with mascarpone whisked together with fresh orange juice

curry me up

Let's clear up a myth here: peanut butter is really good for you and not something unhealthy that only kids like. This feast will provide you with slow-release energy for extended vitality, circulation-boosting spices from the curry and lots of bone-building calcium and immune-boosting bugs from the yogurt.

- Peanut Butter Pick-Me-Up, *see* page 138
- Curried Fish with Rice & Peas, *see* page 128
- Live yogurt topped with runny honey and pistachio nuts

cheeky chicken

Of all the perceived luxury foods, smoked salmon is the best nutritional value for money. It has protein, vitality-boosting essential fatty acids and lots of vitamin D. With more protein, blood-building iron, energy-generating zinc from the chicken and slow-release energy and potassium from the bananas, there will be no stopping you after this feast.

- Organic smoked salmon on organic wholemeal bread with lemon and black pepper
- Nutty about Chicken, *see* page 132
- Baked bananas, split and filled with dark-chocolate buttons

mine's a pint

With betacarotene and energy-giving fruit sugars in the melon and the lightest of egg-based dessert on either side of the stew, this is a well-balanced vitality feast. Apart from masses of muscle-building protein in the beef, you get the benefit of all the energizing B vitamins from the beer.

- Slices of ogen melon
- Beer Stew, *see* page 135
- crème caramel, preferably homemade

plum gorgeous

It's a fallacy that you have to eat meat for strength and vitality. This veggie feast will be welcomed by true vegetarians and enjoyed by even the most committed carnivores. With energy-boosting ingredients in each course, it's a perfect meal if you're feeling at your lowest ebb.

- Bruschetta of slices of wholemeal bread smeared with garlic, topped with a slice of tomato and a slice of avocado, then put under a grill for 3 minutes
- Spicy Veggie Stew, *see* page 127
- Halved, stoned plums stewed gently in red wine with half a stick of cinnamon for 20 minutes, then served with live yogurt

figgy lamb feast

Sorrel is a greatly undervalued leaf. Similar to spinach, it's winter-hardy and can provide vitality-boosting nutrients throughout the year. Followed by these wonderful braised lamb shanks with lentils, which provide energy and strength-building protein, and ending with figs, this meal is truly a feast of super-vitality.

- Auntie Leiki's Sorrel Soup, *see* page 126
- Lamb, Lentil & Carrot Casserole, *see* page 136
- Fig Fantasy, *see* page 133

aphrodisiac

smoked mackerel soup

serves
4

Yes, it does sound strange to put porridge with smoked fish, but this unusual combination tastes great. There's slow-release energy from the oats, protein from the fish, and the leeks and onion add not only flavour but enormous amounts of protective phytochemicals.

4 tablespoons olive oil
2 large onions, finely chopped
2 leeks, finely chopped
1 garlic clove, finely chopped
1 large carrot, finely chopped
1 large potato, grated
500ml or 18fl oz fish stock
4 fillets smoked mackerel (not canned)
55g or 2oz unsalted butter
115g or 4oz porridge oats
4 tablespoons double cream

1 Put the oil into a large saucepan and sweat the vegetables for about 10 minutes.
2 Add the stock and another 500ml or 18fl oz freshly boiled water and simmer for 15 minutes.
3 In another pan, poach the mackerel fillets with the butter and just enough water to cover them for 6 minutes.
4 Flake the fish. Add it to the vegetable mixture along with the poaching liquid.
5 Stir in the oats and leave to stand for 10 minutes.
6 Pour into bowls and serve with a spoonful of cream on each.

RICH IN Essential fatty acids from the mackerel, B vitamins and soluble fibre from the oats, vitamin E from the olive oil, betacarotene from the carrots

buckwheaties

Buckwheat isn't a real cereal. In fact, the plant is related to rhubarb. It's extremely rich in a natural chemical called rutin, which keeps the inner lining of blood vessels clear and healthy. This circulatory stimulant combined with vitamin E, essential for sexual function, makes this a very sexy dish.

225g or 8oz buckwheat flour
1 beaten egg
1 tablespoon brown caster sugar
2 teaspoons ground cinnamon
About 300ml or 10fl oz semi-skimmed milk
85g or 3oz unsalted butter
4 large dessert apples, cut into rings
2 tablespoons sesame seeds

1 Mix together the flour, egg, sugar and cinnamon with enough of the milk to make a smooth batter.
2 Heat the butter gently.
3 Dip the apple rings in the batter, then sauté in the butter until crisp.
4 Serve with the sesame seeds scattered on top.

RICH IN Rutin, from the buckwheat flour, which strengthens blood vessels and helps prevent chilblains and broken veins, circulation-friendly properties from the cinnamon, calcium from the milk, vitamin C from the apples, and protein and vitamin E from the sesame seeds

casanova's delight

I don't like oysters at all, but I love watching other people's obvious delight as they feast on these magnificent molluscs. Oysters are the richest natural source of the mineral zinc, which is essential for male sexual function. Just remember that Casanova ate seventy a day – usually in the bath with his latest paramour.

175ml or 6fl oz dry white wine

1 tablespoon light soy sauce

1 tablespoon runny honey

1 tablespoon capers, soaked for 5 minutes in milk, drained and lightly crushed

2 teaspoons dried dill or fennel

6 flat, round native oysters

280g or 10oz thin salmon fillet, skin removed, cut into bite-sized chunks

1 small bunch of seedless black grapes

1 bunch of watercress

1 Mix together the first five ingredients.

2 Warm through and allow to cool.

3 Prise open the oysters and add their liquid to the sauce.

4 Spoon the sauce over the salmon and the oysters and leave to marinate in fridge for 2 hours.

5 Serve on a bed of watercress, garnished with the grapes.

RICH IN Zinc from the oysters, essential for a great sex life; a good balance of omega-3 and omega-6 fatty acids from the salmon; nourishing and strengthening properties from the grapes; vitamin C and iron from the watercress (sex and anaemia don't make good bedfellows)

sage & nut burgers

Although I'm not a vegetarian, many of my friends are. It's not a problem when they come over for supper; I just make these lovely burgers using the sage which grows in our herb garden all year round and the remains of the crusts of wholemeal bread which we put into a blender, freeze and make into breadcrumbs. So simple!

225g or 8oz mixed unsalted nuts
115g or 4oz wholemeal breadcrumbs
1 onion, finely chopped
About 200ml or 7fl oz olive oil
300ml or 10fl oz low-salt vegetable stock
6 fresh sage leaves, roughly torn
4 tablespoons wholemeal flour

1 Put the nuts and breadcrumbs into a food processor and grind until fine.
2 Sauté the onion gently in 2 tablespoons of the oil until soft but not brown.
3 Tip in the ground nut mixture and the stock and mix until smooth.
4 Stir in the sage leaves.
5 Shape into four burger patties.
6 Dust with the flour.
7 Heat the rest of the oil and shallow-fry the burgers until crisp: about
  4 minutes each side.

RICH IN Protein, vitamin B and magnesium from the nuts, anti-cancer agents from the onion, heart-protective contents in the olive oil, phytoestrogens from the sage, to balance female hormones

mango tango

This is the ultimate loving cup. Mangos and avocados are a huge source of vitamin E: an essential nutrient for a sparkling love life. The beetroot not only colours this soup a romantic pink but is a renowned blood tonic. And the final touch is the delicate flavour of coriander, known throughout Asia as a gentle and long-acting aphrodisiac.

1 large organic Hass avocado, stone and skin removed, cut into chunks
1 large organic mango, stone and skin removed, cut into chunks
250ml or 9fl oz organic beetroot juice
200ml or 7fl oz bio-yogurt
2 tablespoons coriander leaves, very finely chopped

1 Blend first 4 ingredients in a food processor.
2 Pour into a saucepan and heat just to simmering point.
3 Serve sprinkled with coriander leaves.

RICH IN Heart-protective mono-unsaturated fats from the avocado, protective antioxidants from the mango, anti-cancer and anti-ageing substances in the beetroot juice, digestion benefits from the coriander

fantasy flan

Asparagus, the favourite of all European fantasy foods, is one example of the truth matching the folklore. Extremely rich in potassium, folic acid and the natural plant chemical asparagine, asparagus is particularly helpful for men wanting to have a good sex life. The boost to blood flow from cayenne and the vitamin E from sesame seeds are the icing on the cake.

1 sheet ready-made puff pastry
20–24 asparagus tips
2 small eggs
200ml or 7fl oz fromage frais
½ teaspoon cayenne pepper
1 tablespoon sesame seeds

1 Lay the pastry in a greased 20cm (8in) flan tin.
2 Arrange the asparagus in a cartwheel, with the green tips facing the rim.
3 Beat the eggs into the fromage frais. Stir in the cayenne pepper.
4 Pour the mixture over the asparagus. Sprinkle with sesame seeds.
5 Bake at 220°C or 425°F or gas mark 7 for 25 minutes.

RICH IN Purines, from the asparagus, which are great to help relieve rheumatism and arthritis – but don't eat it if you've got gout; zinc and vitamins A, B, D and E from the eggs

dame barbara's beef

Many people ridiculed her for her ostentatious style, but my dear friend the late Dame Barbara Cartland, who I'd been privileged to know for nearly forty years, was one of the sexiest women I've ever met – even when she was in her 90s. She often said that red-blooded men need lots of red meat in their diets. She was right, so here's the perfect recipe.

115g or 4oz chopped walnuts
Half a garlic clove, peeled and finely chopped
Half a can of anchovies, drained, soaked in milk for 10 minutes,
  then drained again
1 teaspoon Tabasco sauce
4 tablespoons peanut or rape-seed oil
2 x 200g or 7oz organic beef fillet steaks, 1cm (½ inch) thick

1 Whizz the walnuts, garlic, anchovies, Tabasco and 1 tablespoon of the oil in a food processor.
2 Sear the steaks in the rest of the hot oil for 10 seconds each side.
3 Press the nut mixture into the steaks. Leave in fridge for half an hour, then bake at 200°C/400°F/gas mark 6 for 20 minutes.

RICH IN Conjugated linoleic acid from the beef (as long as it's organic) which helps fight cancer; protein and slow-release energy from the walnuts; garlic to help beat heart disease and many types of inflammatory conditions, essential fatty acids from the anchovies

pan-fried trout

serves
4

The great twentieth century song writers captured the essence of the vital link between mood and romance with songs like 'I'm in the Mood for Love'. Food is part of this mysterious, eternal conundrum. Loving food must add to the ambience – and this simple, light dish is guaranteed to bring on the romance.

1 small onion, finely chopped
1 small garlic clove, finely chopped
4 tablespoons olive oil
1 teaspoon each paprika and chilli powder
400g or 14oz can chickpeas, thoroughly washed
200g or 7oz can chopped tomatoes
4 pink salmon trout fillets
Lemon slices and fresh coriander for garnish

1 Sweat the onion and garlic in half the oil for 5 minutes.
2 Stir in the paprika and chilli powder and cook for 2 minutes.
3 Add the tomatoes and chickpeas and simmer until tender: about 10 minutes.
  Add more water if the mixture starts to dry out. Mash the chickpeas roughly.
4 Pan-fry the trout fillets in rest of oil for 2 minutes each side.
5 Put the chickpea mash on plates, top with the fish, garnish with lemon
  slices and coriander.

RICH IN Essential fatty acids from the fish, circulatory-boosting substances from the spices, heart-protective properties from the onion and garlic, phytoestrogens from the chickpeas, blood-protective agents from the lycopene in the tomatoes

chicken pesto

This is a truly romantic dish. The starch in the rice encourages the release of mood-enhancing tryptophan from the brain, and the high vitamin E content of pine kernels in the pesto is extremely important for a healthy sex life. Here's a simple-to-prepare recipe, which is light and easy to digest.

115g or 4oz basmati rice
Half a green pepper, deseeded and very finely diced
3 spring onions, very finely diced
55g or 2oz unsalted butter
4 tablespoons red pesto, shop-bought or make your own
2 skinned chicken breasts

1 Cook the rice according to the packet instructions, with pepper and
   onions added halfway through cooking time.
2 Mix the butter into the pesto and rub into the chicken breasts.
3 Grill the chicken breasts for 8 to 10 minutes each side.
4 Put rice on plates and drizzle with any stirred surplus sauce from the chicken.
5 Arrange the chicken breasts on top.

RICH IN Protein and easily absorbed iron and zinc from the chicken; volatile oils, which aid digestion and are strongly mood-enhancing, from the basil in the pesto; complex carbohydrates, which stimulate the release of emotion-triggering tryptophan in the brain, from the rice; vitamin C from the green pepper

sexy stir-fry

All shellfish and seafood are credited with aphrodisiac qualities. This is partly due to the fact that they're rich in zinc, which is essential for male sexual function, but also I think they're nearly always eaten with fingers: a sensual act in itself.

3 spring onions, cut diagonally
1 large garlic clove, finely sliced
1 small red chilli, deseeded and finely chopped
1cm or ½ inch fresh ginger root, peeled and grated
About 5 tablespoons stir-fry oil
3 heads pak choi, quartered lengthwise
8 broccoli florets
16 raw king prawns
1 tablespoon freshly squeezed lime juice
2 tablespoons light soy sauce
2 tablespoons finely chopped coriander leaves

1 Sweat the spring onions, garlic, chilli and ginger in half the stir-fry oil.
2 Add the pak choi and broccoli and stir until wilted.
3 In another pan, stir-fry the prawns in more oil until pink all over, about 5 minutes.
4 Tip the prawns into the vegetable mixture and warm through for 1 minute, stirring continuously.
5 Stir in the lime juice and soy sauce.
6 Sprinkle with the coriander leaves to serve.

RICH IN Vitamin B_{12} from the prawns, antioxidants from the spring onions and garlic, aphrodisiac power from the coriander, vitamin C from the pak choi and lime juice

almond bananas

Just the dish to finish a romantic meal, this is a banana split for adults only. There's loads of potassium in the bananas to protect you from cramp at inappropriate moments, the mysterious flavour of cardamom, which is widely regarded as an aphrodisiac in the Far East, and the heady aroma of sweet almonds from the amaretto.

2 teaspoons ground cardamom

85ml or 3fl oz orange juice

50ml or 2fl oz lemon juice

2 tablespoons caster sugar

3 tablespoons morello cherry jam

25g or 1oz butter

4 bananas, peeled and split lengthwise

3 tablespoons amaretto

4 tablespoons flaked almonds

1 Mix together the first six ingredients in a small saucepan and warm through over a low heat.

2 Put the bananas in an ovenproof dish, arranging them to fit snugly.

3 Pour the amaretto over the bananas, then pour over the warmed mixture.

4 Sprinkle with the flaked almonds and cook at 180°C or 350°F or gas mark 4 for 20 minutes.

RICH IN Potassium, vitamin B_6 and folic acid from the bananas, vitamin C from the orange and lemon juice, circulation-boosting substances from the cardamom, heart-protective mono-unsaturated fats from the almonds

raspberry ripe

The popular drink *granita*, a bit like a half-frozen lemon sorbert, is served at practically every café around the Mediterranean. Add fresh raspberries, not only the most romantic of fruits but abundant in essential minerals, and the sweet crispness of *langues du chat* biscuits and you have a deliciously light dessert guaranteed to create that loving feeling. Never underestimate the powerful aphrodisiac appeal created by attractive fruits such as raspberries.

55g or 2oz caster sugar
Juice of 4 unwaxed lemons
350ml or 12fl oz mineral water
1 punnet raspberries
4 *langues du chat* biscuits

1 In a small saucepan, dissolve the sugar in the water and lemon juice. Cool.
2 Pour the mixture into a freezer-proof container.
3 Freeze for 2 hours, breaking up the crystals every 30 minutes.
4 Put four raspberries in the bottom of two Champagne glasses or tall sundae dishes. Fill with the *granita* mixture. Top with the rest of the fruit and serve with the biscuits on the side.

RICH IN Vitamin C and bioflavonoids from the lemons, more vitamin C and cardiovascular protective substances from the raspberries

quick romantic drinks

If romance is on your mind, then it's easy to make the perfect fresh-fruit cocktail. Juice 115g or 4oz each of blueberries and raspberries with 225g or 8oz each strawberries and stoned cherries. The colour is the epitome of romance and the vitamins and minerals have just what you need to induce those wonderful warm and amorous feelings. If you really want to push the boat out, top up with Champagne for the best fizz you've ever drunk – I call it Beds Fizz (after the county, of course!).

Alternatively, for the natural equivalent of Viagra in a glass, try making an Eastern Promise by juicing 2 fresh figs, 225g or half a pound black grapes, and one pawpaw. Top up with pink Champagne and sip as an aperitif. The sacred fig tree of India has been worshipped for 5,000 years and the Spartan athletes of ancient Greece were fed a diet rich in figs, to improve their performance – and not just in the arena. Add the noblest of fruits, the grape, which is both cooling and aphrodisiac, and the oriental aroma of pawpaw, and you have a juice that is full of eastern promise.

Whatever you do, go easy on the booze. A little wine, or better still, Champagne, will work wonders. But don't forget the infamous Brewer's droop, or as Shakespeare warns men more subtly in *Macbeth*, 'Drink provokes the desire, but it taketh away the performance.'

romantic feasts

bean feast

Beans may not be the first food that springs to mind when you think of romantic meals, but you'd be wrong to dismiss them. They're full of phytoestrogens, hormone-like substances which help balance women's hormones. Together with the circulatory boost from buckwheat, this menu will do more than you can imagine for your love life.

- Smoked Mackerel Soup, *see* page 143
- Bean salad made with a mixture of canned beans, sliced onions, hard-boiled eggs and vinaigrette dressing mixed with mayonnaise
- Buckwheaties, *see* page 144

oyster special

In folklore, there are no more trusted aphrodisiacs than coriander, oysters and almonds. Add carrots so that you can see in the dark, salmon to protect the heart and bananas to prevent inopportune cramp.

- Carrot and coriander soup – use your own recipe or buy a good organic variety
- Casanova's Delight, *see* page 145
- Almond Bananas, *see* page 153

beef beauty

Wherever mangoes grow, they're revered as healing and sensuous fruits. Beef up your man with Britain's greatest culinary contribution, and then melt his heart with raspberries. Who could resist?

- Mango Tango, *see* page 147
- Dame Barbara's Beef, *see* page 149
- Raspberry Ripe, *see* page 154

performance power

The traditional English starter of potted shrimps belies its appearance. These tiny brown creatures are a powerhouse of protein and mineral energy. They're followed by light, vegetarian burgers, for stamina and healthy hormones, and this feast finishes with calcium-rich cheese and grapes for instant energy.

- Potted shrimps with wholemeal melba toast
- Sage & Nut Burgers, *see* page 146
- Camembert cheese with wholemeal bread and grapes

chickpea out

Here we are with finger food again – and if you've no idea what makes them sensuous and sexy, rent the video of *Tom Jones* (the movie, not the singer). The mushy peas in this trout recipe are, in fact, chickpeas, which have been included for their hormonal benefits. And finally, you can feed each other with some delicious strawberries.

- Asparagus with melted unsalted butter
- Pan-fried Trout, *see* page 150
- Strawberries scattered with black pepper and sprinkled with balsamic vinegar

garlic

protective

rosemary

olive oil

bright eyes

Bearing in mind that many of us spend most of our days sitting in front of VDUs and that age-related macular degeneration (AMD), a progressive eye disease, is the most common cause of blindness in the elderly, this juice is designed specifically to protect the eyes of people of all ages. But don't think of it just as a healthy preventative – it's delicious, too.

4 carrots, top and tail removed, and peeled if not organic
1 bunch of watercress
1 handful of spinach leaves
1 small handful of parsley
2 kale leaves

1 Reserving a few sprigs of parsley, put all the ingredients through a juicer.
2 Chill slightly and serve with the reserved parsley floating on top.

RICH IN Eye-protective vitamin A and betacarotene from the carrots; other carotenoids, lutein and xeathine, which specifically protect against AMD, from spinach and kale; vitamin C from the watercress; diuretic properties from the parsley

traditional white onion soup

The French, of course, have hijacked dark onion soup with cheese-crusted bread and called it their own. This softer, smoother version with a lovely creamy look and texture is a traditional winter protector in East Anglia. Because its main ingredient is onions, you couldn't have a more protective start to a meal or lunch treat.

3 large white Spanish onions, halved, then very finely sliced
55g or 2oz, unsalted butter
2 tablespoons flour
700ml or 1¼ pints full-fat milk
1 bouquet garni
2 bay leaves
12 peppercorns
150ml or 5fl oz cream, yogurt or crème fraîche
Half a handful of finely chopped parsley leaves

1 Sweat the onions very gently in the butter until soft but not brown.
2 Stir in the flour, mix well and cook for 3 minutes, stirring continuously, until the mixture is well-combined and starts to thicken.
3 Pour in the milk and stir well.
4 Add the bouquet garni, bay leaves and peppercorns and simmer very gently, stirring occasionally, until the onions are soft – about 15 minutes.
5 Remove the bouquet garni, bay leaves and peppercorns.
6 Stir in the cream, yogurt or crème fraîche. Warm through if necessary.
7 Serve with the parsley scattered on top.

RICH IN Protective and antibacterial chemicals from the onions, antiviral essential oils from the bouquet garni, circulatory stimulants from the peppercorns, bone-protective calcium from the milk

mussel power

This is such a simple dish and incredibly easy to prepare. Although shellfish are known mostly for their romantic effects, they're also hugely protective because of their high zinc content. And the other ingredients add to the health benefits.

2kg or 4^1/$_2$ lbs mussels, washed and scraped; discard any that
   don't close when tapped
25g or 1oz unsalted butter
1 garlic clove, finely chopped
3 spring onions, finely chopped
^{1}/$_2$ teaspoon dried oregano
1 glass white wine
4 tablespoons curly parsley, finely chopped

1 Put the mussels into a very large saucepan. Cover and heat until all shells are open and the liquid has drained out. Discard any that are still closed.
2 Strain the liquid through a piece of muslin and reserve.
3 Put the butter, garlic, onions and oregano into the pan and sweat gently for 2 minutes.
4 Add the reserved liquor, wine and 1 glass of water. Stir for another minute. Add the mussels, cover and boil briskly for 5 minutes.
5 Empty into a large bowl and sprinkle with the parsley to serve.

RICH IN Heart-protective chemicals from the garlic and onions, vitamin A and C from the parsley, zinc and essential fatty acids from the mussels

lentil mania

In my view, pulses of all descriptions should be part of everyone's daily diet. They're packed with protein, simple to prepare and very sustaining – which is particularly important if you're living on a low budget. Here, I've cooked them with tuna, carrots and spring onions. Eat some fresh fruit afterwards and you couldn't have a more balanced and protective meal.

115g or 4oz lentils
3 large spring onions, finely chopped (including green part)
3 tablespoons olive oil
1 egg
150ml or 5fl oz milk
175g or 6oz can of tuna, drained
1 medium carrot, grated
55g or 2oz flaked almonds

1 Boil the lentils in water, stirring occasionally, until tender – about 20 to 30 minutes.
2 Over a gentle heat, soften the onion in the oil.
3 Beat the egg into the milk.
4 Combine the tuna, lentils, onions and egg mixture. Place in a shallow casserole dish.
5 Scatter with the almonds. Bake at 200°C or 400°F or gas mark 6 for 30 minutes.

RICH IN Slow-release energy and protective phytoestrogens from the lentils, protein from the tuna and almonds, cell-protective carotenoids from the carrots, B vitamins from the eggs, calcium from the milk

quick quiche

serves
4–6

To many people, quiche still brings back memories of the 1970s, when it was THE meal to have at lunchtime. They weren't wrong. This easy recipe is quick to make, delicious to eat and easily digested – perfect if you haven't got the appetite to face a heavy meal and your immune system needs a boost.

1 sheet of ready-made shortcrust pastry, baked blind for 15 minutes
   in a 25cm or 10in flan case
4 tablespoons extra-virgin olive oil
1 small onion, thinly sliced
Half a red and half an orange pepper, deseeded and cut into small cubes
1 small courgette, thinly sliced
1 tablespoon each dried marjoram and thyme
2 eggs
225g or 8oz mascarpone cheese
25g or 1oz Parmesan cheese, grated
150ml or 5 fl oz plain bio-yogurt

1 Heat the oil and sweat the onion, peppers and courgettes. Add the marjoram and thyme and continue cooking gently for 2 minutes.
2 Beat eggs, the add the mascarpone, Parmesan and yogurt.
3 Put the vegetables into the prepared pastry case. Pour the egg and cheese mixture over them.
4 Bake at 200°C or 400°F or gas mark 6 for 30 minutes.

RICH IN Vitamin C and protective carotenoids from the peppers, essential oils from the thyme and marjoram, protein and calcium from the cheese

spinach chowder

What could be more soothing than a bowl of hot soup: a traditional comfort and resistance-building food, particularly on a cold evening? But this soup has lots more than the comfort factor going for it. If you can't get green lentils, it would work well with any pulse, but make sure you look at the cooking instructions carefully. Some need soaking overnight and boiling for longer.

1 medium onion, chopped

3 garlic cloves, finely chopped

4 tablespoons olive oil

25g or 1oz butter

$1/2$ teaspoon herbes de Provence

175g or 6oz tiny green lentils, thoroughly rinsed

650g or 1lb 7oz spinach (or chard), thoroughly washed and roughly torn

1 Soften the onion and garlic in the oil and butter.

2 Add the lentils, herbs and 850ml or $1^1/2$ pints water.

3 Boil briskly for 10 minutes, then simmer for 25 minutes until almost tender.

4 Add the spinach or chard and continue simmering for another 10 minutes.

5 Liquidize if you like, but this soup tastes great left as it is.

RICH IN Nerve-nourishing B vitamins from the pulses, hormone-balancing plant chemicals from the sage in the herbes de Provence, antioxidants from the oregano in the herbes de Provence, heart-protective properties from the olive oil

blueberry beef

Fillet of beef *is* expensive – especially if it's organic. But you don't (and shouldn't) have it every day, so this is a recipe for special occasions. You can rest assured that you're getting a cornucopia of protective nutrients from every ingredient in this dish.

1 large celeriac, peeled and diced
1 medium swede, peeled and diced
2 tablespoons extra-virgin olive oil
2 tablespoons olive oil
2 fillet steaks, preferably organic
2 tablespoons blueberry conserve
A little port or robust red wine

1 Simmer the celeriac and swede together until tender.
2 Drain thoroughly, put back on a gentle heat to dry out.
3 Mash well with the extra-virgin olive oil and keep warm.
4 Heat a griddle pan until very hot. Brush the steaks with a little olive oil and cook oiled side down.
5 Brush again with a little more oil and turn over. How long you cook each side depends on your personal preference.
6 Reserving as much of the juices as possible, put the steaks on hot plates.
7 Turn down the heat in the pan, add the blueberry conserve and scrape in any residues of the meat.
8 Add enough port or wine to give you a thinnish sauce.
9 Serve the beef on the vegetable mash with the sauce poured on top.

RICH IN Protein, iron, B vitamins and minerals from the beef, plus cancer-fighting conjugated linoleic acid if it's organic; cancer-fighting chemicals in the blueberries; fibre, carotenoids and vitamin C from the root vegetables; heart-protective agents from the oils

lamb with anchovies

serves
4–6

When I was first served this recipe by our American friend Sarah I thought it sounded totally contrived. Then I took a mouthful… The anchovies add a certain sweetness which, surprisingly, doesn't taste the slightest bit fishy. They make a wonderful partner for the rather robust but delicious flavour of rosemary.

1 organic shoulder of lamb
55g or 2oz well-seasoned flour
55g or 2oz can of anchovies, drained
6 to 10 small sprigs of rosemary

1 Wash the lamb, dry thoroughly, remove any excess fat and rub all over with seasoned flour.
2 Using a sharp knife, make incisions at equal distances all over the meat.
3 Push one anchovy and a sprig of rosemary into each hole.
4 Turn the oven to its hottest temperature setting. Put in the meat, then turn the heat down immediately to 190°C or 375°F or gas mark 5.
5 Roast for 25 minutes per 450g (1lb) plus 25 minutes extra. Allow to rest for 15 minutes, covered with foil, before carving.

RICH IN Digestion-enhancing and memory-protective properties from the rosemary; protective essential fatty acids from the anchovies; iron, zinc, protein and B vitamins from the lamb

bread salad

Whenever I'm in Spain, I always order some variation of this salad wherever I am; every tapas bar, café or restaurant seems to have its own. The difference between most of theirs and my exclusive creation is the addition of eggs and basil, which add to the protective nutrition of this dish.

2 garlic cloves, very finely chopped
4 thick slices of coarse wholemeal bread, crusts removed and cut into
   1cm or half-inch cubes
3 tablespoons olive oil
4 tomatoes, quartered
1 red onion, finely cubed
1 red pepper, finely diced
1 cucumber, peeled and sliced
6 hard-boiled quails eggs, or 2 hard-boiled hens eggs, sliced
Juice of 1 lemon
Extra-virgin olive oil for drizzling
Small handful of fresh basil leaves

1 Sauté the garlic and bread in the olive oil until the bread is crisp.
2 Drain on kitchen paper and put into a large bowl.
3 Add the tomatoes, onion, red pepper, cucumber, eggs and lemon juice
   and toss well.
4 Drizzle with a little extra-virgin olive oil.
5 Tear the basil leaves and scatter over the salad to serve.

RICH IN Protein, B vitamins, vitamin E, minerals and fibre from
the bread; cancer-fighting lycopene from the tomatoes; vitamin C
from the pepper, cucumber, tomatoes and lemon; heart-protective
chemicals from the oils

rose-scented fruits

Dried fruits aren't only tremendously nutritious and protective, they're the height of convenience, too. In fact, apart from the yogurt or cream, this beautiful-to-look-at and wonderful-to-taste dessert is a real store-cupboard star.

250g or 9oz ready-to-eat prunes (Californian are best for this dish)
250g or 9oz ready-to-eat dried apricots
300ml or 10fl oz rosewater
White wine
Live yogurt

1 Arrange the prunes and apricots attractively in a large, shallow, lightly buttered ovenproof dish.
2 Pour over about three-quarters of the rosewater.
3 Add enough white wine just to cover the fruit.
4 Cover with aluminium foil and bake at 180°C or 350°F or gas mark 4 for 20 minutes.
5 Mix the rest of the rosewater with the yogurt and pour over the fruit to serve.

RICH IN Protective antioxidants from the prunes; gut-protective fibre, betacarotene and heart-protective potassium from the apricots; calcium and gut-protective, immune-boosting good bacteria from the live yogurt

quick protective soups

Easy to make and perfect for lunch at home, or at work or school in a thermos.

spicy garlic soup

Provides B vitamins from the bread and all the goodness of garlic.

10 chopped garlic cloves

1 chopped onion

3 tablespoons olive oil

1 teaspoon crushed aniseeds

Two slices stale wholemeal bread

Sweat the garlic and onion in oil until golden. Add the aniseeds and stir for 1 minute. Add 1 litre or 1¾ pints of water, bring to boil and simmer 10 minutes. Add the bread and simmer for 10 minutes, or until the soup thickens.

leek and potato

This thick, nourishing soup makes a perfect protective meal.

1 garlic clove, chopped

55g or 2oz butter

2 leeks, chopped

350g or 12oz small new potatoes, unpeeled and quartered

1 large onion, sliced

850ml or 1½ pints vegetable stock

2 tablespoons finely chopped fresh parsley

freshly ground pepper

150ml or 5fl oz double cream

Sweat the garlic in the butter. Add the leeks, potatoes and onions and cook for 10 minutes. Add the stock and simmer for 20 minutes. Liquidize. Add the parsley, pepper and cream.

protective feasts

mad about lentils

To prevent and alleviate chest infections, no food is better than onion soup. Eaten together in this meal with hormone-regulating lentils and vitamin C-rich oranges, it's a perfect winter combination.

- Traditional White Onion Soup, *see* page 160
- Lentil Mania, *see* page 162
- Peeled, sliced oranges sprinkled with a little orange brandy

quichefest

This is a meal for all seasons as the ingredients are available throughout the year. It's an all-round protective medley and hugely practical, as you can make enough of each dish at one time to produce two meals.

- Spinach Chowder, *see* page 164
- Quick Quiche, *see* page 163
- Baked apples stuffed with dried fruit

blueberry hill

All shellfish and seafood are powerful health-protectors, and this surf-and-turf meal will set you up with almost a week's worth of immune-boosting nutrients. Even the chocolate mousse makes you feel good and may reduce the pain of arthritic joints because of the chocolate's theobromine, a natural anti-inflammatory.

- Oysters *au naturel* with lemon OR a plate of king prawns with lemon and wholemeal bread
- Blueberry Beef, *see* page 165
- Organic chocolate mousse, preferably homemade

lovely lamb

Here's a meal to protect your eyesight, boost blood and muscles and build strong bones. You may think that cheesecake has no place in a healthy cook book, but you'd be wrong. We all need treats, and this one provides both calcium and pleasure.

- Bright Eyes, *see* page 159
- Lamb with Anchovies, *see* page 166
- Lemon cheesecake, preferably homemade

show your mussels

The Moorish influence in southern Spain isn't just in the buildings; it has also left its indelible mark on the regional cooking. Bread salads are a staple in the Middle East, dried fruits are part of their culinary history and rosewater is as widely used in their desserts as ketchup is on burgers in the West.

- Bread Salad, *see* page 167
- Mussel Power, *see* page 161
- Rose-scented Fruits, *see* page 168

pick-me-up

wide awake juice

The zingy flavour of cinnamon, mixed with the smoothness of peanut butter and yogurt is enough to make anyone feel good. This smoothie is the perfect start to a hectic day and wonderful if you're recovering after an illness or just feeling a bit under the weather.

2 apples
1 pear
2 bananas
1 tablespoon smooth peanut butter
100ml or 3½ fl oz plain bio-yogurt
½ teaspoon cinnamon

1 Put the first three ingredients through a juicer.
2 Pour the juice into a bowl and beat in the peanut butter and yogurt.
3 Serve with the cinnamon scattered on top.

RICH IN Instant energy from the fruit sugar in the apples and pear, slower-release energy from the banana, good carbohydrates from the peanut butter, volatile oils from the cinnamon

beet soup

serves
3–4

If you're feeling sleepy and lethargic, there's nothing better than a nourishing soup to get you on your feet again. The great thing about this recipe is that it tastes equally delicious made in the evening, chilled overnight and drunk as a juice in the morning.

1 onion, finely chopped
3 tablespoons rape-seed or peanut oil
3 small uncooked beetroot, peeled and very finely diced
2 English apples, peeled, cored and cut into quarters
¼ Savoy cabbage, finely sliced
850ml or 1½ pints stock, preferably homemade

1 Sweat the onion in the oil. Add the beetroot and soften gently for 20 minutes.
2 Mix in the apples, most of the cabbage and the stock.
3 Simmer until the vegetables are tender – about 25 minutes.
4 Stir in the reserved cabbage leaves and serve.

RICH IN Antioxidants from the onion, blood-cleansing properties from the beetroot, antibacterial sulphur from the cabbage, heart and circulation protection from the apples

spiced scramble

This is a very versatile dish, which is equally delicious for brunch, lunch, afternoon tea or a light supper. The best way to cook it is to leave the egg mixture until it starts to set, then, using a palette knife, begin to push it in gently from the sides so that you can still see the difference between the white and the yolks. Organic and free-range eggs are an essential choice for this recipe, as there's virtually zero risk of salmonella.

2 tablespoons unsalted butter
½ teaspoon turmeric
2 small courgettes, grated
5 organic, free-range eggs, lightly beaten
2 teaspoons freshly chopped parsley

1 Heat the butter and gently fry the turmeric for 2 minutes.
2 Stir in the courgettes and cook for 1 minute.
3 Pour in the beaten eggs and cook, folding occasionally, until they're lightly scrambled.
4 Serve with the parsley scattered on top.

RICH IN Protein, zinc and vitamins A,B,D and E from the eggs, circulation-boosting and cancer-fighting properties from the turmeric, essential oils from the parsley, vitamin C from the courgettes

wake-me-up chicken

If you really need to be on your toes, there isn't a better combination than onions, chicken and the traditional herbs of the bouquet garni: sage, rosemary, thyme, chervil. This is the perfect antidote for the treatment of FAIFOT Syndrome: Falling Asleep in Front of the Telly.

3 tablespoons virgin olive oil
1 onion, finely chopped
1 garlic clove, chopped
350g or 12oz boned, skinned chicken breasts, cut into thin goujons
150ml or 5fl oz chicken or vegetable stock, preferably homemade
55g or 2oz mushroom, sliced
55g or 2oz green beans, cut into 2.5cm or 1-inch batons
1 bouquet garni
250ml or 9fl oz mixed double cream and crème fraîche

1 Heat the oil and gently sweat the onion and garlic.
2 Add the chicken pieces and stir-fry gently until golden.
3 Stir in the stock, mushrooms and beans. Add the bouquet garni.
4 Continue cooking, covered, on the hob for about 15 minutes, or until the meat and vegetables are tender.
5 Pour off any excess liquid. Remove the bouquet garni. Add the crème fraîche and cream to serve.

RICH IN Low-fat protein, plus easily absorbed iron and zinc from the chicken, vitamin B_6 from the breast of the chicken, antioxidants from the onion and garlic, immune-boosting natural chemicals in the mushrooms

couscous shrimps

Shellfish are great if you need a boost but don't really feel like eating a heavy meal. They're light, easy to digest and quick to cook. In this recipe I've teamed them with couscous, a wonderful source of energy – and you don't need much time to make it.

280g or 10oz couscous
8 spring onions, finely chopped
Handful of chives, snipped finely
Half a medium cucumber, peeled, deseeded and cut into julienne strips
8 cherry tomatoes, quartered
225g or 8oz shrimps, cooked, shells removed
8 tablespoons of your favourite vinaigrette dressing
3 tablespoons lemon juice

1 Wash the couscous thoroughly. Simmer in water for 20 minutes, stirring occasionally. Drain and allow to cool slightly.
2 Pour into a large bowl and add next 5 ingredients. Mix thoroughly.
3 Stir in the vinaigrette, then the lemon juice.
4 Serve with warm wholemeal pitta bread.

RICH IN Carbohydrates from the couscous, vitamin E and zinc from the shrimps, stimulating natural chemicals from the chives, cancer-fighting lycopene from the tomatoes

caperble salmon

You couldn't get a simpler meal than this. It takes less than ten minutes to prepare and is heaving with goodness. Chervil, a greatly under-used herb in my opinion, gives it a very distinctive flavour of mild aniseed. And capers, with their spicy sweetness, are one of my favourite cooking ingredients.

315g or 11oz thick salmon fillet, skinned

4 tablespoons rape-seed oil

115g or 4oz mange-tout, simmered for 5 minutes, torn into 2.5cm or
   1-inch chunks, drained but kept warm

2 plump lettuce hearts, cut into quarters and thoroughly washed

1 tablespoon capers, soaked in milk for 5 minutes, then drained

1 hard-boiled egg, roughly chopped

95ml or 3¼ fl oz warm fish or vegetable stock, preferably homemade,
   infused with 3 sprigs chervil, half a well-crushed garlic clove and
   3 finely chopped spring onions

95ml or 3¼ fl oz vinaigrette dressing

1 Brush the salmon fillet with the oil. Grill for 6 minutes each side.

2 Arrange the lettuce and mange-tout in a serving dish.

3 Put the fish chunks on top and scatter with the capers and egg.

4 Mix the warm stock and vinaigrette together and pour over
   the salad to serve.

RICH IN Vitamin C and energizing coumarins from the chervil, circulation-boosting chemicals from the capers, essential fatty acids from the salmon, protein from the egg

blueberry pineapples

The wonderful colours, delicious flavour and health-packed ingredients in this scrumptious recipe make it a real winner. Use it as the perfect start to the day, an impressive starter or a palate-cleansing dessert.

2 thick slices fresh pineapple, cores removed
1 punnet blueberries
115g or 4oz mixed crushed seeds and nuts
4 tablespoons runny honey

1 Arrange the pineapple slices on an ovenproof plate.
2 Fill each core area with blueberries.
3 Scatter the nuts and seeds on top.
4 Drizzle with the honey.
5 Put under a hot preheated grill for 3 minutes.

RICH IN Healing enzymes and energy-giving fruit sugar from the pineapple, cancer-fighting chemicals from the blueberries, protein from the nuts, antibacterial properties from the honey

leek & rocket soup

Vichysoisse is, of course, a traditional soup which almost reeks of the peasant cuisine of France and its earthy flavours of potatoes teamed up with leeks. Here I've added another touch, rocket, which gives that wonderful peppery taste. If you've got a garden, grow it yourself rather than paying the extortionate price charged in supermarkets. It's a weed and grows like a weed. I defy anyone to be able to kill it.

2 leeks, trimmed and finely sliced
55g or 2oz unsalted butter
3 medium potatoes, peeled and cubed
850ml or 1½ pints vegetable stock
1 large handful of rocket
150ml or 5fl oz live yogurt

1 Sauté the leeks gently in the butter until soft but not brown.
2 Add the potatoes and stir until covered with the butter.
3 Pour in the stock, bring to the boil, then simmer until the potatoes are soft – about 15 minutes.
4 Cool slightly, then liquidize with the rocket.
5 Warm gently and serve with a spoonful of yogurt on top.

RICH IN Detoxifying chemicals from the leeks, fibre and vitamins B and C from the potatoes, healthy gut-protective bacteria from the yogurt, cleansing and analgesic volatile oils from the rocket

quick beef stir-fry

Stir-fries are one of the easiest ways of cooking. They take just minutes and taste great. Be sure that you trim off all the excess fat from the beef and try, if possible, to buy organic meat. It contains a special type of natural fat called conjugated linoleic acid, which helps fight cancer and stimulates the conversion of fat into energy.

400g or 14oz lean steak, cut into thin strips
1cm or ½ inch fresh ginger root, grated
1 garlic clove, finely chopped
2 tablespoons light soy sauce
4 tablespoons sesame oil
115g or 4oz mange-tout, trimmed
1 small red pepper, deseeded and cubed
1 small glass of dry sherry

1 Put the beef, ginger, garlic and soy sauce into a large bowl. Mix well and leave to marinate for about 30 minutes.
2 Heat the oil in a wok.
3 Add the beef mixture and fry until just turning brown.
4 Tip in the mange-tout and red peppers and stir-fry for another 4 minutes.
5 Pour in the sherry and warm through before serving.

RICH IN Protein, iron, B vitamins and minerals from the beef, warming and antiseptic properties from the ginger, antioxidants from the garlic, vitamin C and betacarotene from the mange-tout and red peppers

dracula juice

serves
2

This may sound like a rather unappetizing combination, but believe me, it tastes good. As well as the garlic warding off vampires, this juice is great for soothing sore throats and helping recovery from coughs, colds or flu.

2 garlic cloves, peeled
1cm or ½ inch fresh ginger root
4 apples, quartered but unpeeled
2 celery sticks, preferably with leaves

1 Reserving some of the celery leaves, put all the ingredients through a juicer.
2 Serve with the celery leaves floating on top.

RICH IN Cancer-fighting ellagic acid from the apple, antioxidants from the garlic, circulation-boosting coumarins from the celery, stimulating chemicals from the ginger

spicy meatballs

The beauty of this dish is that it can be made with the leftovers of the Sunday roast. It's equally delicious hot or cold, makes wonderful party or picnic food and survives well packed into the kids' lunchboxes.

1 onion, finely chopped
55g or 2oz fresh pine kernels
450g or 1lb minced lamb, fresh or previously cooked
5 large mint leaves, finely chopped
2 eggs

1 Put the onion and pine kernels into a food processor and whizz until smooth.
2 Add the lamb, mint and egg and mix well.
3 Using your hand, mould the mixture into small ball about the size of a walnut, then flatten slightly.
4 Put under a hot grill and cook for 2 minutes each side.

RICH IN Protein, iron and B vitamins from the lamb, digestive volatile oils from the mint, vitamin E from the pine kernels, zinc and vitamins A, B and D from the egg

rabbit & prune stew

Yes, they do look sweet and cuddly, but the truth is that man has been eating rabbits since we were living in caves. The real news is that they have amazing nutritional benefits. In this recipe, which comes from Tuscany, they're cooked with prunes, which gives the meat a wonderfully sweet flavour and makes the whole dish a real health treat.

1 onion, finely chopped
2 garlic cloves, finely chopped
4 tablespoons olive oil
1 rabbit, jointed
3 tablespoons wholemeal flour
200ml or 7fl oz red wine
12 prunes, stones removed
3 bay leaves

1 Soften the onion and garlic in the oil and remove from the pan.
2 Roll the rabbit in the flour, add to the pan and brown all over.
3 Put back the onion and garlic, add the wine, prunes and bay leaves.
4 Bring to a boil and simmer for an hour or until the meat is tender, adding more wine (or water) if it looks as if it's drying out.

RICH IN Antioxidants from the prunes, the richest cancer-fighting food you'll find; virtually fat-free protein from the rabbit; more antioxidants from the red wine; digestion-stimulating volatile oils from the bay leaves

pick-me-up diets

Traditionally, all recipe books used to contain a section on cooking for convalescents and invalids, and it saddens me that this is no longer the case. So unless you've got some of your grandmother's old cookery books, here are some ideas for superfoods to choose when you need a pick-me-up after illness.

Breakfast should include: porridge; yogurt with honey and pine kernels; melon; soaked dried fruits with yogurt and cinnamon; wholemeal toast; boiled, poached or scrambled eggs.

For lunch, try white fish, oily fish, broccoli, spinach, carrots, free-range chicken, rosemary, thyme, garlic and sage.

Evening meals should consist of light salads, soups made with root vegetables, barley, millet, fruit salads with almonds, low-fat cheeses and avocados.

Extras treats: fresh fruit, especially grapes, dates, kiwi-fruit, citrus fruits and berries; unsweetened fresh fruit juices; vegetable juices; dried fruit; fresh nuts and seeds.

Obviously, exact nutritional needs will depend on the nature of any illness, but the general principles are to include easily digestible, nutrient-rich, appetizing and easy-to-eat foods. The antioxidant vitamins A, C and E, protective minerals like zinc, and a high intake of iron to ensure good haemoglobin, are essential. As a general guide, eat plenty of the following foods: blackcurrants, berries, citrus fruits and kiwi fruit, which are all rich in vitamin C and bioflavonoids. Dates contain iron and easily converted calories. Oats provide protein, B vitamins, calcium, potassium and magnesium. Fish are full of easily digested protein and minerals. Root vegetables, broccoli, carrots all contain healing betacarotene. Dried fruits provide energy. Garlic, cinnamon, sage, rosemary and thyme contain antiseptic and circulation-stimulating properties.

Cut down on: refined carbohydrates, sugars, alcohol, high-bran foods, animal fats and red meat.

pick-me-up feasts

here's to you, chuck

This whole meal is a tonic on a plate. Garlic, chicken, honey and blueberries are some of Nature's most restorative foods.

- Dracula Juice, *see* page 182
- Wake-Me-Up Chicken, *see* page 176
- Live yogurt topped with honey and blueberries

couscous special

This meal is a real *entente cordiale*. What could be more Italian than bruschetta, more north African than couscous or more English than strawberries and cream? A geographical medley of vitality foods that are also highly protective.

- Bruschetta made by grilling slices of wholemeal baguette, smearing them with halved cloves of garlic, topping with a slice of avocado, then tomato, then mozzarella cheese and grilling until the cheese melts
- Couscous shrimps, *see* page 177
- Strawberries and cream

fish fantastic

All the traditional blood-strengthening components of beetroot, easily digestible fish and bone-building cheese make this delicious meal perfect after any illness or injury – especially if you've sustained a fracture.

- Beet Soup, *see* page 174
- Caperble Salmon, *see* page 178
- Cheese with oat cakes

lively lamb

Cretan men are the longest-lived in Europe, and what could be more redolent of southern Greece than rocket, koftas and fresh figs? This meal is awash with anti-ageing nutrients.

- Leek & Rocket Soup, *see* page 180
- Spicy Meat Balls, *see* page 183
- Fresh figs

stir-fried in minutes

The Far Eastern diet is renowned for its anti-cancer and restorative properties, and there can be few homes nowadays that don't boast a wok in the kitchen. This combination of body-building stir-fried beef, super-nourishing avocado, protective blueberries and healing pineapple makes this a real three-star pick-me-up meal.

- Tomatoes stuffed with a mixture of mashed avocado, cottage cheese and caraway seeds
- Quick Beef Stir-Fry, *see* page 181
- Blueberry Pineapple, *see* page 179

calming

cool as a cucumber

Cucumber has been used in the Ayurvedic medicine of India for thousands of years because of its calming and soothing properties. It doesn't really taste of much, but when combined here with the delicious sweetness of pineapple and the vibrant colour of strawberries, it makes a wonderfully relaxing put-your-feet-up smoothie.

15cm or 6in cucumber
4 apples
1 small pineapple, prickly leaves removed
1 medium bunch flat-leaf parsley
125ml or 4fl oz live yogurt
2 plump strawberries, cut into quarters

1 Put the first four ingredients through a juicer.
2 Mix in the yogurt.
3 Top with the strawberry quarters.

RICH IN The enzyme bromelain from the pineapple, which aids digestion and speeds healing after any injury; vitamin C and antiviral benefits from the strawberries; soluble fibre from the apples; gut-protective bacteria from the yogurt

packed with power

serves
4

Most people think of pears as a fruit you put on the dining room table to look good and make other people think you eat healthily. That's totally wrong as they have many nutritional benefits. In this juice they're given an even greater boost with the apples, kiwi fruit and celery. Just what you need when your body needs a lift but your brain is telling you to slow down

2 Conference pears, quartered but not peeled
3 kiwi fruit, halved but not peeled
2 apples, preferably the English Cox variety, quartered but not peeled
2 celery sticks, with leaves if possible, cut into large chunks
3 fresh mint leaves, plus 2 extra, finely chopped, as a garnish

1 Put all the ingredients through a juicer.
2 Mix until well-combined.
3 Chill thoroughly.
4 Serve with the extra chopped mint on top.

RICH IN Soluble fibre from the apples, vitamin C from the kiwi fruit, calming chemicals from the celery, potassium and more fibre from the pears

treat yourself to tofu

This is a really relaxing vegetarian treat that is brimming with wonderful flavours and good nutrition. The interesting taste comes from the oils and other ingredients in which the tofu is marinated – an essential process as tofu doesn't have much flavour of its own. If you don't like the texture of tofu – and you eat meat – this dish works equally well with cubes of chicken breast.

200g or 7oz tofu
30ml or 1fl oz soy sauce
30ml or 1fl oz balsamic vinegar
2 tablespoons walnut oil
1 tablespoon crushed capers
1 tablespoon runny honey
1 pack prepared stir-fry vegetables
4 tablespoons safflower oil
115g or 4oz rice noodles or fine spaghetti, cooked as per
   packet instructions

1 Cut the tofu into bite-sized cubes. Mix together the next five ingredients
   and use half to coat the tofu.
2 Bake tofu at 220°C or 425°F or gas mark 7 for 15 minutes, stirring occasionally.
3 Stir-fry the vegetables in the safflower oil for 4 minutes.
4 Add the tofu and rest of the sauce, turn down the heat and warm through.
5 Serve the tofu mixture on rice, noodles or spaghetti.

RICH IN Calming plant hormones from the soya, traditionally
soothing benefits from the honey, calming carbohydrates
from the rice or pasta, vitamin C from the vegetables

porridge & kipper soup

serves
3–4

I was on holiday on the Isle of Skye when I first saw this dish offered on a menu. Quite honestly, I thought it sounded disgusting. I was persuaded to try it, though, and it tasted wonderful. Whenever we make it at home, it always brings back memories of heather-covered hillsides and the mist coming in over the Irish Sea…

2 large onions, finely chopped

2 leeks, washed and finely chopped

1 garlic clove, finely chopped

1 floury potato, peeled and grated

1 fat carrot, grated

2 tablespoons olive oil

55g or 2oz unsalted butter

4 skinned kipper fillets

85g or 3oz fine porridge oats

2 generous tablespoons double cream

1 Sweat the onions, leeks, garlic, potato and carrot gently in the oil and half of the butter for 15 minutes.
2 Pour in 850ml or 1½ pints water and simmer for a further 15 minutes.
3 Meanwhile, poach the kipper fillets in water and the rest of the butter for 6 minutes.
4 Flake the kippers and add to the soup, along with the porridge oats.
5 Leave to stand, covered, for at least 10 minutes and serve with a dollop of cream in each bowl.

RICH IN Mood-soothing ingredients from the oats, a good balance of omega-3 and -6 fatty acids from the kipper, protective plant chemicals from the garlic, leeks and onions, calcium from the cream

192 S U P E R F E A S T

herb & onion tart

serves
4–6

Yes, this dish does contain egg yolks, butter and double cream. But when your stress levels have reached screaming point, you deserve a bit of spoiling and self-indulgence. This smooth and creamy dish – accompanied by a glass of decent wine and a crisp salad – will certainly do the trick.

700g or 1lb 9oz mixed red and white onions, cut into very fine rings
60g or 2¼ oz unsalted butter
3 tablespoons freshly chopped oregano or marjoram leaves
1 sheet shortcrust pastry, baked blind for 10 minutes in a 23cm or
   9-inch flan tin
3 organic egg yolks
6 tablespoons double cream

1 Soften the onions very gently in the butter. Cover and continue simmering for 15 minutes.
2 Chop the oregano or marjoram leaves. Add to the onions and simmer for 15 minutes more.
3 Pour the onion mixture into the prepared pastry case.
4 Mix together the egg yolks and cream. Season to taste with salt and pepper. Pour over the onion mixture and bake at 190°C or 375°F or gas mark 5 for 25 minutes.

RICH IN Heart-protective chemicals from the onion, volatile oils from the oregano and marjoram, protein from the eggs, calcium from the cream

spiced chicken

Salads are extremely helpful if you're feeling under pressure, haven't eaten much during the day because you've been too busy and want something light but nutritious in the evening. If you know you won't have much time to prepare meals, make a big bowl of this wonderful salad and keep it, covered, in the fridge for two or three days. It also make a good dish to take on a picnic.

1 tablespoon garam masala
300ml or 10fl oz good mayonnaise
350g or 12oz cooked and shredded chicken
85g or 3oz cooked rice
1 small red onion, very finely chopped
2 tender celery sticks, very finely chopped
115g or 4oz diced red, yellow or green peppers
125ml or 4fl oz vinaigrette dressing
3 kiwi fruit, peeled and cut into chunks

1 Mix the garam masala into the mayonnaise.
2 Combine the chicken, rice, onion, celery, and peppers, and pour on the vinaigrette.
3 Leave the mayonnaise and the salad to marinate for at least an hour.
4 Mix the mayonnaise into the salad and gently fold in the kiwi fruit, being careful not to break them up.

RICH IN Vitamin C and bioflavonoids from the kiwi fruit, anti-stress spices from the garam masala, carbohydrates and peace-inducing tryptophans from the rice, vitamin C and betacarotene from the peppers

hunky dory

It has to be said that John Dory isn't the most attractive-looking fish, but it tastes delicious. It's not always easily available, but if you can't find it, red mullet will do equally well. The ancient tale maintains that the black spot on each side of a John Dory are the fingerprints of St Peter – and this is certainly a dish blessed with health benefits.

4 tablespoons extra-virgin olive oil
2 tablespoons lemon juice
1.3kg or 3lb John Dory, filleted
2 tablespoons breadcrumbs
½ teaspoon dried oregano

1 Mix the oil and lemon juice together. Stir in the breadcrumbs and oregano and season to taste with salt and pepper.
2 Rub the mixture over the fish and leave it to marinate in the fridge for 1 hour.
3 Drizzle the fish with oil and grill under a medium heat for 10 to 15 minutes each side.

RICH IN Protein and minerals from the fish, heart-protective natural chemical from the olive oil, mood-enhancing (and reputedly aphrodisiac) volatile oils from the oregano

dish stress

Liver is an absolute godsend to anyone who needs to get stress and anxiety levels down. Cooked here with grapes, a storehouse of aromatic compounds, and you have the perfect – and quickly prepared – end to a busy day.

2 spring onions, very finely chopped
1 small garlic clove, very finely chopped
3 tablespoons extra-virgin olive oil
175g or 6oz chicken livers, membranes removed and cut into large chunks
55g or 2oz flour seasoned with salt, pepper and 1 teaspoon paprika
115g or 4oz white seedless grapes, peeled if you can be
   bothered, and halved
4 slices of bread taken from a wholemeal baguette
1 small bunch of parsley, finely chopped

1 Soften the onions and garlic in the oil.
2 Roll the liver pieces in the seasoned flour, add to the onion/garlic pan, turn up the heat, and cook for 3 minutes, stirring constantly, until seared.
3 Add about half a cup of almost boiling water and simmer for 1 minute, scraping the pan thoroughly.
4 Take off the heat and mix in the grapes. Leave for 1 minute.
5 Serve on lightly toasted bread, scattered with parsley.

RICH IN Vast amounts of vitamins A and B from the liver, vitamin C from the grapes, heart protection from the onions and garlic

duck delight

Duck has always seemed to me an ideal comfort food. Although I love a traditionally roasted Aylesbury duck – which used to be bred exclusively in the countryside where I now live – it is quite fatty and really only part of a healthy diet if you eat it just occasionally. In this recipe, I've used only the duck breasts and added herbs and spices which add more flavour and nutritional benefits.

½ teaspoon ground coriander
1 teaspoon allspice
85ml or 3fl oz live yogurt
Half a bunch each coriander and flat-leaf parsley, finely chopped
2 duck breasts, with skin
3 tablespoons rape-seed oil

1 Mix together the herbs, spices and yogurt.
2 Smear all over duck portions, pushing some of the mixture under the skin. Leave in the fridge for 2 hours.
3 Drizzle the duck breast with oil and roast at 180°C or 350° F or gas mark 4 for 20 minutes.
4 Turn up heat to 220°C or 425°F or gas mark 7 for 10 minutes to crisp the skin.

RICH IN Protein, iron, zinc and nearly all the B vitamins from the duck – but delicious though it is, don't eat all the skin; cleansing and mood-enhancing properties from the coriander; gut-protective good bacteria from the yogurt; diuretic qualities from the parsley

sardine kedgeree

serves
3–4

This is an unusual variation of traditional kedgeree and a far cry from the dish associated with the days of the Raj. It's packed with flavour and goodness and works well with fresh fillets of any oily fish: mackerel, herrings or pilchards, for example. This is a particularly good dish for women as it's rich in essential fatty acids for emotional balance, as well as vitamin D and calcium for strong bones.

2 eggs, beaten
55g or 2oz cooked rice
115g or 4oz Cheddar cheese, grated
350g or 12oz sardine fillets, skinned
675g or 1½ lbs baby spinach

1 Mix together the beaten eggs, rice and half the cheese.
2 Put half the mixture in an ovenproof dish.
3 Place the fish on top.
4 Cover with the rest of the mixture.
5 Scatter the remaining cheese on top and bake at 200°C or 400°F or gas mark 6 for 35 minutes.

RICH IN Protein, iron, zinc, essential fatty acids and vitamin D from the sardines, folic acid from the spinach, complex carbohydrates from the rice, calcium from the cheese

brandy apricots

Flambéed dishes are show-off time. They may look very difficult when you see them cooked at a table in an expensive restaurant, but believe me, they're not that complicated to cook at home – and they do add a smile to the end of the day. This one tastes just gorgeous.

70g or 2½ oz caster sugar
125ml or 4fl oz red wine
3 tablespoons lemon juice
2 star anise
25g or 1oz butter
6 ripe apricots, left whole
3 tablespoons apricot brandy

1 Heat the sugar with the wine, lemon juice and star anise.
2 Add the butter and stir over a gentle heat until it melts.
3 Put the apricots into the liquid, cover and poach for 15 to 20 minutes or until just tender.
4 Heat the apricot brandy. Set it alight and pour over fruit.
5 Serve with double cream.

RICH IN Betacarotenes from the apricots, vitamin C from the lemon juice, heart-protective chemicals from the red wine, the calming volatile oil estragol from the star anise

rice & prune pud

This pud doesn't have a skin to fight with, and the additional benefits of prunes (or any other dried fruit) make it a soothing dessert for the end of the day. The high natural sugar content of dried fruit keeps the blood sugar supply to the brain on an even keel, which is emotionally relaxing. Tryptophan in cheese and the lethargy-fighting components of cinnamon turn this into the most peaceful pud around.

100g or 3½ oz pudding rice
1 teaspoon lemon juice
40g or 1½ oz sugar
700ml or 1¼ pints milk
115g or 4oz pitless prunes, snipped
2 tablespoons mascarpone cheese
1 teaspoon cinnamon

1 Put the rice, lemon juice and sugar in a saucepan. Add about 200ml or 7fl oz water and simmer until the water is nearly absorbed.
2 Pour in the milk and simmer for 10 minutes.
3 Add the prunes and continue simmering for 20 minutes, stirring occasionally, until rich and creamy.
4 Serve with a dollop of mascarpone and sprinkled with cinnamon.

RICH IN Cancer-fighting chemicals from the prunes, calcium from the milk and mascarpone, vitamin C from the lemon juice, antiviral essential oils from the cinnamon

quick stress-busting drinks

If you're feeling stressed and anxious try camomile or lime blossom. They're both available commercially in tea bags; simply add boiling water, cover, leave for five minutes and add a little honey.

If insomnia's your problem, valerian or hops make an ideal nightcap, particularly if you add some honey as above. Both these herbs are very calming and help you to relax and so get off to sleep more easily. Ideally they should be drunk half an hour before bedtime and sipped slowly.

If it's indigestion that's keeping you awake – and it is one of the most common causes of insomnia – then use a few sprigs of fresh mint, a teaspoonful of dried mint or a commercial mint tea bag. The essential oils in mint are the best of all antacids and will soon settle your stomach.

For mood swings that are associated with the menstrual cycle, juice two or three apples, a stick of celery, a handful of parsley and three sage leaves, and stir into half a glass of soya milk. The sage and soya milk help regulate hormone levels and the diuretic effect of parsley and celery gets rid of the uncomfortable swellings which many women suffer – and which adds to their monthly anxiety.

anti-stress feasts

chicken special

Just getting into the kitchen is a great way to beat stress. With the right attitude and enough time, cooking is an absorbing and relaxing pastime. The bonus with this relaxing meal is that the chicken dish will keep for a day or so, so you needn't cook tomorrow.

- Porridge & Kipper Soup, *see* page 192
- Spiced Chicken, *see* page 194
- A bowl of satsumas

that's cool

Please don't turn your nose up at the prunes, as they deserve far more than their reputation as a laxative. Weight for weight, they contain more heart- and cancer-fighting chemicals than any other food.

- Cool as a Cucumber, *see* page 189
- Herb & Onion Tart, *see* page 193
- Rice & Prune Pud, *see* page 200

laid-back liver feast

Anyone who's stressed needs extra B vitamins to nourish the nervous system and these simple chicken livers provide them all. Starting with pink grapefruit, which is rich in betacarotenes, and finishing with calcium-rich goat cheese, this a light and nourishing meal.

- Pink grapefruit
- Dish Stress, *see* page 196
- Soft goat cheese with lychees and wholemeal crackers

fish treat

All fish are a source of iodine, often in short supply in modern diets. This essential mineral is needed by the thyroid gland, which controls your metabolism. If it's not working efficiently, you feel tired, sluggish and stressed.

- Packed with Power, *see* page 190
- Hunky Dory, *see* page 195
- Fresh fruit salad

delicious duck

The calming and mood-enhancing properties of basil in the starter sets the tone for this feast. The combination of yogurt and sweet allspice in the duck is typically Middle Eastern and goes perfectly with the flavour and texture of vitamin B-rich duck breast.

- Tomato, onion and basil salad
- Duck Delight, *see* page 197
- Brandy Apricots, *see* page 199

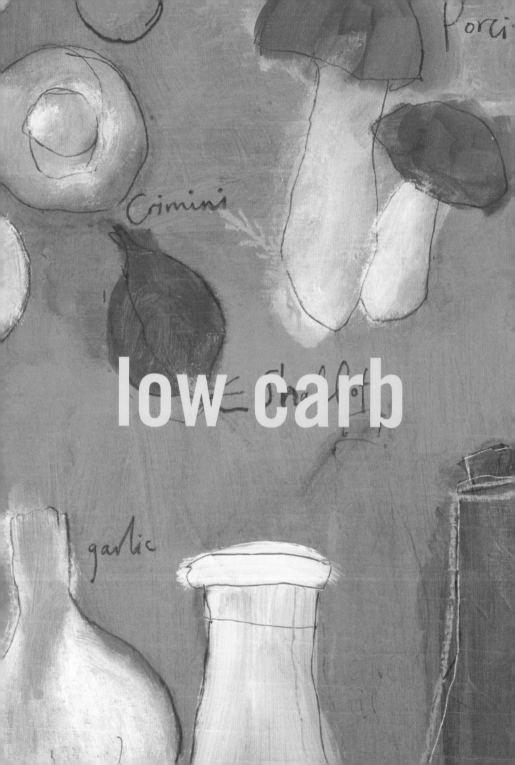

low carb

4-fruit juice

I'm a great fan of fresh juices as a way of getting enormous amounts of nutrients in a relatively small amount of food. This one looks and tastes absolutely wonderful.

4 nectarines or peaches
1 pear, unpeeled
Half a lemon, peeled
10 plump strawberries
2 small sprigs of mint

1 Stone the nectarines or peaches.
2 Put all the ingredients through a juicer.
3 Pour the juice into two tall glasses.
4 Decorate with the mint sprigs to serve.

RICH IN Vitamin C from all the ingredients, potassium from the pears, pectin (soluble fibre) from the strawberries, digestive properties from the mint

herb & vegetable juice

Since juicing and juice bars exploded into British cuisine, there seems no end to the variations you can make. This is one of the most popular in our home as it combines the benefits of vegetables with the health-giving properties of some of my favourite herbs.

6 sage leaves
2 teaspoons freshly chopped rosemary leaves
4 carrots, tops and tails removed and peeled unless organic
3 celery sticks, preferably with leaves
1 handful parsley leaves

1 Put all the ingredients through a juicer, reserving a few parsley leaves.
2 Pour into tall glasses.
3 Decorate with reserved parsley.

RICH IN Betacarotene from the carrots, diuretic properties from the celery and parsley, cleansing and antiseptic natural chemicals in the sage

fresh tomato soup

This delicious and light soup is ideal as a first course on a summer's day or as a light lunch any time of the year. It has a wonderfully fresh aroma and flavour – with hardly a calorie in sight.

1 medium onion, very finely chopped
2 garlic cloves, very finely chopped
3–4 tablespoons olive oil
6 large tomatoes, peeled and quartered
850ml or 1½ pints vegetable stock, preferably homemade
4 teaspoons pesto

1 Sauté the onion and garlic gently in the oil.
2 Tip in the tomatoes and simmer gently until mushy.
3 Pour in the stock and cook for 5 minutes.
4 Season and allow to cool slightly.
5 Serve with a spoon of pesto floating on top.

RICH IN Heart protection from the onions and garlic, cancer-fighting lycopene and vitamin C from the tomatoes, volatile oils from the basil in the pesto

spiced spinach soup

This fusion soup combines the benefits of spinach, often associated with northern climates, and the hot eastern appeal of chilli and coriander. It's perfect if you're on a low-carb diet – not for too long, I hope, as it really isn't healthy – but if your friends aren't on one, too, serve the soup with garlic or cheese croutons on top.

1 onion, very finely chopped
1 garlic clove, very finely chopped
4 tablespoons olive oil
Half a small red chilli, seeds removed and very finely chopped
Half a handful each of chopped coriander, parsley and mint, leaves only
450g or 1lb fresh spinach, chopped
1litre or 1¾ pints vegetable stock, preferably homemade
200ml or 7fl oz crème fraîche

1 Sauté the onion and garlic gently in the oil until soft but not brown.
2 Stir in the chilli, coriander, parsley and mint and continue cooking, stirring, for 2 minutes.
3 Add the spinach and about a cup of the stock and cook for 3 minutes, still stirring, until the spinach starts to wilt.
4 Pour in the rest of the stock and simmer for 10 minutes.
5 Stir in the crème fraîche to serve.

RICH IN Heart-protective chemicals from the onion and garlic, volatile oils in the chilli, digestion-promoting agents in the coriander and mint, folic acid and cancer-fighting carotenoids from the spinach

mushroom & red lettuce salad

This unusual warm salad has plenty of eye appeal as well as great flavour. The contrast of dark mushrooms and the red lettuce and tomato is deliciously combined with the opposing textures of these health-giving ingredients. As a starter, lunch or light supper, this is an ideal autumn and winter salad.

12 medium flat mushrooms
3 tablespoons olive oil
2 garlic cloves, finely chopped
1 red lettuce, such as radicchio, divided into leaves
4 tomatoes, sliced
About 115g or 4oz Parmesan cheese

1 Grill the mushrooms for a minute on both sides.
2 Tip into a frying pan with the oil and garlic and sauté gently.
3 Divide the lettuce among four plates.
4 Arrange the tomato around the outside.
5 Put three mushrooms on each pile of lettuce.
6 Drizzle over the garlic olive oil.
7 Shave the Parmesan with a potato peeler and scatter on top.

RICH IN Protein, phosphorus and potassium from the mushrooms, vitamin C and lycopene from the tomatoes, calcium from the Parmesan cheese, heart-protective chemicals from the garlic

turkey with anchovy sauce

Turkey shouldn't be left just for Christmas. It's now extremely economical and has hardly any fat. This dish uses turkey breasts cold, so they're excellent for picnics, buffet parties or as a side dish at summer barbecues.

1 carrot, chopped

1 celery stick,chopped

1 onion, finely sliced

1 tablespoon white-wine vinegar

2 turkey breasts

2 anchovy fillets

A little milk

1 hard-boiled egg

2 tablespoons finely chopped parsley

Extra-virgin olive oil

1 Put the carrot, celery, onion and vinegar into a pan of hot salted water. Bring to the boil and simmer for 3 minutes.

2 Add the turkey breasts and continue to simmer gently for 45 minutes.

3 Leave the breasts to cool in the stock.

4 Soak the anchovy fillets in a little milk for 3 minutes to remove the salt.

5 Chop the egg and put into a blender with the anchovies, parsley and enough oil to make a creamy sauce.

6 Remove the breasts from the stock (keep the stock for other recipes.

7 Slice the breasts and serve with the sauce on top.

RICH IN Protein, iron and zinc from the turkey, essential fatty acids from the anchovy, lecithin and more protein from the eggs, diuretic and digestive properties from the parsley

lamb with peppers

Cook this relatively quickly prepared dish and, thanks to the evocative smells of onion and garlic, your kitchen will be transported to somewhere in southern Spain or Italy. You'll also share some of the health benefits of the Mediterranean diet.

1 medium onion, finely chopped
2 garlic cloves, finely chopped
4 tablespoons olive oil
550g or 1¼ lb lean lamb fillet, cubed
1 red pepper, deseeded and sliced
1 yellow pepper, deseeded and sliced
1 x 400g or 14oz can tomatoes
2 large sprigs fresh rosemary

1 Sweat the onion and garlic in the oil until soft but not brown.
2 Remove the onion and garlic with a slotted spoon and add the lamb fillet to the oil remaining in the pan.
3 Fry, stirring constantly, until golden all over, then remove.
4 Return the onion and garlic to the pan, add the peppers, tomatoes and rosemary and bring to a boil.
5 Simmer gently for 10 minutes.
6 Return the lamb and simmer for another 5 minutes.
7 Remove the rosemary and check the seasoning.

RICH IN Heart-protective properties from the onion and garlic, cholesterol-lowering chemicals in the garlic, protein from the lamb, vitamin C and betacarotene from the peppers and tomatoes

broccoli & cauliflower au gratin

A variation on an old favourite, when this gratin was made solely with cauliflower and a simple cheese. The broccoli and other unusual ingredients give this dish extra bite, extra flavour and extra colour. They also add huge health benefits without many carbs

450g or 1lb, broccoli, cut into florets
450g or 1lb, cauliflower, cut into florets
2 egg yolks
300ml or 10fl oz milk
175g or 6oz low-fat soft cheese
2 teaspoons mustard seeds
55g or 2oz crushed walnuts
55g or 2oz Emmental cheese, grated

1 Steam the broccoli and cauliflower for about 7 minutes, until the vegetables are just turning soft.
2 Beat the egg yolks into the milk. Bring slowly to a boil, stirring continuously.
3 Remove from the heat and add the soft cheese, mustard seeds and half the walnuts.
4 Arrange the broccoli and cauliflower florets alternately in an ovenproof dish.
5 Pour over the sauce, sprinkle with the rest of the walnuts, then the Emmental cheese.
6 Put under a hot grill until the cheese bubbles.

RICH IN Cancer-fighting carotenoids from the broccoli, folic acid from the cauliflower, calcium and vitamins A and B from the cheeses, antioxidant essential fatty acids from the walnuts

sardines with mustard sauce

This healthy Mediterranean favourite is hardly ever cooked in this country. That's a shame because sardines are amazingly nutritious, extremely cheap, widely available and very quick to cook. I've paired them here with a sauce that takes less than a minute to make.

12 sardines, cleaned and gutted

Olive oil

8 tablespoons plain live low-fat yogurt

2 teaspoons Dijon mustard

1 Brush the fish with the oil.

2 Line a grill pan with foil.

3 Put the fish into the pan and heat the grill until very hot.

4 Grill the fish for 2 minutes each side.

5 Mix together the yogurt and mustard.

6 Serve the fish with the sauce on the side.

RICH IN Protein, iron, zinc and vitamin D from the sardines, cholesterol-lowering properties from the olive oil, calcium and good gut bacteria from the yogurt

chicken with thyme & lemon

serves
4

This is another quick dish which goes well with a variety of accompaniments. A simple salad is ideal if you're on a low-carb kick, but friends may like rice or new potatoes boiled in their jackets as well. This dish also cooks perfectly on a barbecue.

6 tablespoons olive oil
Juice of 2 lemons
2 garlic cloves, finely chopped
2 large sprigs fresh thyme
4 chicken breasts

1 Mix together the first 4 ingredients. Season to taste.
2 Add the chicken breasts and coat with the marinade.
3 Cover and leave for at least an hour – or leave in the fridge overnight.
4 Heat the grill to maximum and cook the chicken breasts for about
   5 minutes each side, basting with the marinade.

RICH IN Vitamin C from the lemons, heart protection from the olive oil and garlic, antiseptic volatile oils from the thyme, protein and vitamin B_6 from the chicken breasts

quick compote

Any sort of compote is really packed with goodness – and the wonderful thing about them is they're so versatile. Most, like this one, would be equally at home at the end of a dinner party, for breakfast the next day or packed up and taken to work for lunchtime.

400g or 14oz ready-to-eat prunes
400g or 14oz other mixed dried fruit, preferably containing blueberries
  and cranberries
2 lemons
2 oranges
3 tablespoons dark rum, brandy or other favourite liqueur
2 tablespoons runny honey

1 Chop all the dried fruit so that it's all the size of a little finger nail.
2 Juice the citrus fruit and mix together with the rum, brandy or liqueur
  and the honey.
3 Pour over the dried fruit mixture and leave to stand for at least 3 hours.

RICH IN cancer-fighting antioxidants from the prunes; more antioxidants if the rest of the dried fruit contains blueberries and cranberries; vitamin C from the citrus fruit; antiseptic healing agents from the honey

happy woman's diet

Crash diets aren't healthy. It's impossible to get all the nutrients needed to lead a normal life. That said, there are situations when people need to lose weight quickly: for example, if they are going into hospital for an operation. And sometimes, of course, losing a bit of weight is vital to a woman's self-esteem. So here's a five-day regime I've used for my patients for years with great success.

DAY 1
Breakfast Half a large melon.
Light meal or snack Vegetable soup or carrot and celery juice. Raw vegetable salad with brown rice and olive oil and lemon juice dressing.
Main meal Mixed salad. Any cooked green vegetables with a can of your favourite beans (but not baked – and rinse them well) and 1 teaspoon olive oil.

DAY 2
Breakfast Freshly juiced apple and carrot or fresh orange.
Light meal or snack The rest of yesterday's soup. Salad, baked sweet potatoes.
Main meal Salad, cooked green vegetables. Cooked cauliflower sprinkled with grated cheese and browned under the grill.

DAY 3
Breakfast Half a grapefruit. Apple. Natural yogurt with a little honey and some chopped nuts.
Light meal or snack Baked potato with butter or 1 tablespoon sour cream and chopped fresh herbs. Coleslaw. A ripe sweet pear.
Main meal Vegetable and cheese casserole: wash and slice 1 green, 1 red and 1 yellow pepper, 2 courgettes, 3 tomatoes, 1 large onion, 2 garlic cloves. Rub a casserole dish with olive oil. Add vegetables in layers, sprinkling each layer with a little olive oil and chopped parsley and basil. Cover with foil. Bake at 180°C or 350°F or gas mark 4 for 45 minutes. Remove foil. Sprinkle with 2 tablespoons grated Parmesan and return to oven until cheese is golden. Serve with steamed broccoli. Orange.

DAY 4

Breakfast **Porridge made with water and 1 tablespoon single cream. One slice wholewheat bread or toast with a little butter.**

Light meal or snack **Winter salad: mix together shredded white cabbage, orange juice, 4 soaked dried apricots and 2 tablespoons of chopped walnuts. Top with a dressing of 2 tablespoons natural yogurt, 2 teaspoons runny honey and grated lemon rind. Stewed apple cooked with cinnamon and cloves.**

Main meal **Watercress Soup. Grilled spiced chicken: allow 1 skinned chicken breast per person and cook extra as this is delicious cold the next day. Chop 1 onion and a garlic clove and put in bowl with some natural yogurt. Heat 1 teaspoon each coriander and cumin seeds for 2 minutes. Crush and add to yogurt with half a teaspoon chilli powder. Pour over chicken and leave for 1 hour. Grill the chicken 10 minutes each side, basting occasionally with marinade. Serve with steamed leeks and carrots.**

DAY 5

Breakfast **Muesli with a sliced banana and a little single cream.**

Light meal or snack **Large baked potato with baked beans. Chicory and watercress salad.**

Main meal **Carrot, ginger and orange soup. Cod with yogurt crust: put a large carton of natural yogurt, 1 chopped onion, 2 cloves peeled garlic, 3 tablespoons coriander seeds, 2 tablespoons fresh mint, 2 teaspoons ground cumin, 2 teaspoons dried dill, 2 teaspoons paprika, plenty of nutmeg and 2 tablespoons chopped parsley into a blender. Put 4 cod fillets into an ovenproof dish. Pour over the sauce and put the fillets under a very hot grill, basting until a crust forms on the fish. Serve with a mixed salad.**

If you haven't cheated you will easily have lost four or five pounds. If you need to lose more, repeat for another five days. Even modest exercise will allow you to eat a bit more, enjoy a couple of glasses of wine a day and the occasional indulgence without putting back those lost pounds.

low-carb feasts

fishy turkey

Turkey isn't just for Christmas. Enjoy it here with an unusual sauce which is also very healthy. Make sure to prepare extra of the Quick Compote; it's great mixed with muesli for breakfast next day.

- 4-Fruit Juice, *see page 205*
- Turkey with Anchovy Sauce, *see page 210*
- Quick Compote, *see page 215*

lamb celebration

This high-protein, low-carb meal is a great example of 'rainbow eating'. The healthiest diet is one that includes foods of as many colours as possible. That's the way to get the widest spread of essential nutrients.

- Fresh Tomato Soup, *see page 207*
- Lamb with Peppers, *see page 211*
- Sliced kiwi fruit and blueberries

thymely chicken meal

It's really worth the effort to use fresh herbs – and even better if you grow your own, as you pick them at their peak and avoid unwanted chemicals. The herbs in these recipes add so much flavour that you can throw away the salt cellar and minimize your risk of high blood pressure.

- Herb & Vegetable Juice, *see page 206*
- Chicken with Thyme & Lemon, *see page 214*
- Good-quality mature Cheddar cheese with Cox or russet apples

when the boat comes in

Parsley, mint, coriander, garlic, and sardines are quintessential flavours of the Mediterranean. This simple low-carb meal is at once energizing, protective and satisfying.

- Spiced Spinach Soup, *see* page 208
- Sardines with Yogurt-Mustard sauce, *see* page 213
- Mixed fresh fruit salad of pawpaws, mangos and pineapple, drizzled with a little honey, and caramelized, if desired

vegetarian style

Nice though they are, vegetarian meals don't have to include high-carb rice, lentils, pasta and potatoes. Here's an entire meal full of vitamins, minerals, protective phytochemicals and, above all, flavour. It's a feast for any carnivore, let alone vegetarians.

- Warm Mushroom & Red Lettuce Salad, *see* page 209
- Broccoli & Cauliflower au Gratin, *see* page 212
- Fresh fruit salad

cleansing

ginger cleanser

'Gingering someone up' has a deep root in herbal medicine. The volatile oil gingerol in ginger is a powerful stimulant to the circulation thus speeding up the expulsion of toxins. This wonderful spice also has a long history in folklore as an aphrodisiac.

4 thick, juicy, clean celery stalks
Half a garlic clove
Scooped out flesh of 3 passion-fruit
400g or 14oz radicchio leaves, thoroughly washed
2 pinches ground ginger

1 Put the first 4 ingredients through a juicer.
2 Pour into 2 glasses and sprinkle with ginger.

RICH IN Diuretic properties from the celery, cholesterol-reducing agents in the garlic, vitamin C in the passion-fruit, circulatory benefits from the ginger

chilled avocado soup

This is one of the prettiest soups you'll find – and as well as being packed with cleansing ingredients, it's also extremely refreshing. It has another advantage if you're entertaining as it can be left in the fridge for a couple of hours before your guests arrive. Don't leave it longer than that, however, or the avocado will start to discolour.

The flesh of 5 large, ripe avocados
1 litre or 1¾ pints vegetable stock, preferably homemade
Juice of 1 lemon
2 garlic cloves, finely chopped
2 red chillies, deseeded and chopped
1 x 200g or 7oz can of organic tomatoes
2 spring onions, roughly chopped
150ml or 5fl oz natural live yogurt
1 heaped teaspoon cayenne pepper
2 tablespoons pumpkin seeds

1 Put the avocados in a blender with the stock, lemon juice, garlic, chillies, tomatoes and spring onions and whizz until smooth.
2 Add the yogurt and cayenne pepper and whizz again.
3 Pour the mixture into a bowl and leave to chill in the fridge.
4 Meanwhile, dry-fry the pumpkin seeds and leave to cool.
5 Serve the soup with the pumpkin seeds scattered on top.

RICH IN Vitamin E and antioxidants from the avocados, circulation-boosting properties from the cayenne and chillies, good gut bacteria in the yogurt, zinc from the pumpkin seeds

veg & chickpea casserole

If you think a healthy casserole probably takes hours to prepare, just look at this recipe. It cooks in little more time than it takes to lay the table and get out the drinking glasses. It's full of nutritional benefits and if you have to persuade kids to take part in your cleansing regime, they'll love it

1 onion, finely chopped
2 large garlic cloves, finely chopped
4 tablespoons olive oil
1 x 400g or 14oz can organic crushed tomatoes
1 x 400g or 14oz can chickpeas
450g or 1lb frozen mixed vegetables
1 bouquet garni
850ml or 1½ pints vegetable stock, preferably homemade
6 basil leaves, roughly torn
1 tablespoon chopped parsley leaves

1 Sauté the onion and garlic in the oil until soft but not brown.
2 Pour in the tomatoes with their juices and bring to a simmer.
3 Drain the chickpeas and rinse thoroughly.
4 Add the chickpeas, mixed vegetables, bouquet garni and stock to the onions and garlic and simmer for 15 minutes.
5 Sprinkle with the torn basil and chopped parsley.

RICH IN Cleansing fibre, B vitamins and minerals that help skin remain healthy and radiant, all from the chickpeas; vitamin C and lycopene from the tomatoes; cleansing volatile oils in the herbs

hungarian chicken

serves
4

Paprika is to the Hungarians what chillies are to the Mexicans. For centuries they've used this mild but cleansing spice to add unique flavours and health benefits to traditional dishes such as goulash and this chicken recipe.

1 teaspoon paprika
2 twists black pepper
Zest and juice of 1 lemon
4 tablespoons rape-seed oil
2 garlic cloves, finely chopped
4 skinless chicken breasts, preferably organic, flattened slightly by bashing them with a rolling pin

1 Mix together the paprika, pepper, lemon, oil and garlic.
2 Put the chicken breasts in a large, shallow bowl. Pour the marinade on top and leave for at least an hour.
3 Remove the chicken from the marinade and cook under a preheated grill for about 7 minutes on each side, until the juices run clear, basting occasionally with the reserved marinade.

RICH IN Good protein from the chicken; vitamin C from the lemon juice; circulation-boosting chemicals from the paprika which help get rid of toxins; heart protection from the garlic

trio carpaccio

Thanks to the growing popularity of Japanese food, the idea of eating raw fish has become increasingly acceptable. This combination of three fish is actually 'cooked' by the marinade, losing none of its nutritious and cleansing properties and making it easy to digest.

225g or 8oz fillet each of fresh salmon, red tuna and sea bass
2 teaspoons capers
4 lemons
4 limes
6 tablespoons best extra-virgin olive oil
3 tablespoons basil leaves, roughly torn
6 sprigs dill, stalks removed

1 Get your fishmonger to slice the fish into paper-thin slices – or put the fillets into the freezer for 30 minutes then slice them yourself.
2 Soak the capers in some milk for 10 minutes to remove the salt, then drain and crush lightly in your fingers.
3 Juice 3 of the lemons and limes.
4 Mix together the oil, fruit juices, crushed capers, basil leaves and dill.
5 Dip each fish fillet in the oil and herb mixture and leave in a wide dish in the fridge for at least 6 hours.
6 Serve garnished with wedges of the extra lemon and lime and chunky wholemeal bread.

RICH IN Vitamin C from the lemons and limes; digestive volatile oils from the dill; iodine from the fish to stimulate the thyroid and speed up the metabolism; anti-inflammatory essential fatty acids, also from the fish

baked cheese & herb polenta

Polenta and rocket: what would we do without those wonderful Italian textures and flavours? But the Italians can't take all the credit; rocket was used in England in Elizabethan times as a tonic. It's so easy to grow – even on the smallest patio – that it makes me mad to see how much they charge for a small pack in a supermarket. This cleansing dish is delish.

1 litre or 1¾ pints herb stock
200g or 7oz coarse polenta
1 large handful of rocket, roughly torn
85g or 3oz Parmesan cheese
2 tablespoons mixed chopped parsley, chervil and chives

1 Bring the herb stock to a boil.
2 Add the polenta gradually, stirring to prevent any lumps.
3 Simmer for about 30 minutes, stirring frequently, until the mixture comes away from the pan.
4 Stir in the rocket, cheese and herbs. Season to taste.
5 Bake in a greased, square dish at 180°C or 350°F or gas mark 4 for 20 minutes, or until firm and golden.

RICH IN Complex carbohydrates in the polenta, protein and calcium in the cheese, blood-purifying properties in the chervil, cleansing diuretic agents in the parsley

cherry bright

I adore cherries. Not only do they look so appealing, they also taste delicious and they're bursting with goodness. This is one of my favourite recipes when English cherries are around for that lamentably short period in the summer. Imported cherries will, of course, do.

1 pack of shortcrust pastry (or homemade)

450g or 1lb fresh red cherries

3 star anise

2 eggs

115g or 4oz ground almonds

115g or 4oz caster sugar

1 Bake the pastry blind in a 23cm or 9-inch flan tin for 10 minutes at 190°C or 375°F or gas mark 5.

2 Stone the cherries and simmer gently in water with the star anise for 5 minutes.

3 Whisk the eggs and mix in the ground almonds and sugar – sieve the latter to prevent lumps.

4 Arrange the cherries in the pastry case. Pour over almond paste. Bake at 200°C or 400°F or gas mark 5–6 for 30 minutes.

RICH IN Vitamin C, potassium cleansing bioflavonoids and cancer-fighting phytochemicals from the cherries; protein, minerals and vitamin E from the ground almonds; cholesterol-lowering lecithin from the eggs; cleansing properties from star anise

fruit terrine

serves
4–6

This delicious dessert is bound to impress, yet it's so simple to make. As with all the recipes in this chapter, it's intended to be easy to digest and perfect for cleansing as an aid to eliminating waste products. Just looking at it will make you want to smile.

2 tablespoons runny honey
2 tablespoons lime or lemon juice
300ml or 10fl oz white wine
Gelatine powder – enough to set just over 300ml or 10fl oz (read the packet)
6 plump strawberries, hulled and cut into 5mm or ¼-inch slices
3 bananas, cut into 5mm or ¼-inch slices
½ teaspoon ground star anise

1 Mix the juice and the wine. Add the honey, stirring until it has dissolved.
2 Sprinkle the gelatine over 4 tablespoons water (or as per instructions)
   until swollen.
3 Line a 450g or 1lb cake tin with clingfilm and arrange the fruit inside it.
4 Pour the gelatine mixture into a small heat-proof container or saucepan
   with the star anise. Warm until completely dissolved.
5 Stir the gelatine mixture into the wine mixture. Pour over fruit. Cover with
clingfilm and leave in the fridge until set.

RICH IN Vitamin C from the strawberries, antibacterial
properties from the honey, pectin and cramp-preventing
potassium from the bananas, cleansing volatile oils from
the star anise

airing cupboard pizza

I was looking for a clean towel when I opened the door to the airing cupboard to find a bowl filled with a lump of dough sitting on top of the clean laundry. 'That's our lunch,' announced my wife. I was just about to suggest that we went to our local pub instead, when she produced this fantastic dish.

450g or 1lb strong white bread flour
1 teaspoon salt
$\frac{1}{2}$ teaspoon sugar
6g or just over $\frac{1}{8}$ oz fast-action yeast
About 75ml or $2\frac{1}{2}$ fl oz olive oil
16 basil leaves
225g or 8oz mixed soft goat cheese (crumbled) and buffalo mozzarella
(finely diced)

1 Whizz the flour, salt, sugar and yeast in a food processor for 30 seconds.
2 With the processor still running, add 3 tablespoons of the oil, then 150ml or 5fl oz warm water until the mixture looks like breadcrumbs.
3 Add another 150ml or 5fl oz warm water, still with the processor running, and whizz until you have a dough. Continue processing for 3 more minutes.
4 Put the dough on a floured board, knead for 2 minutes, brush very lightly with olive oil, cover and keep warm for 1 hour. An airing cupboard is ideal.
5 Bash the dough with your knuckles, divide it into two thin, flat, round pieces and transfer to a greased baking plate. Brush with olive oil and arrange the basil leaves then the cheese on top.
6 Bake at 220°C or 425°F or gas mark 7 for 12 minutes.

RICH IN Cleansing volatile oils from the basil; B vitamins from the flour; mono-unsaturated fats from the olive oil, which help reduce cholesterol; protein and calcium from the cheeses

penne prawn pasta

Pasta must be one of the easiest meals to prepare – and it's such a comfort food. Here I've combined it with a wonderful mixture of herbs, pine nuts, olive oil and Parmesan cheese (the quintessential pesto mixture) and prawns, which are soothing, low-calorie and delicious.

175g or 6oz penne
2 sprigs flat-leaf parsley
20 sprigs basil
3 tablespoons pine nuts
2 garlic cloves
55g or 2oz Parmesan cheese, grated
150ml or 5fl oz extra-virgin olive oil
200g or 7oz cooked, shelled prawns

1 Cook the pasta according to the packet instructions.
2 Put the herbs into a small container of your food processor and whizz for 30 seconds.
3 Add the pine nuts and whizz again. Repeat with the garlic and cheese.
4 Add the oil gradually, whizzing all the time. This completes the pesto sauce.
5 Put the hot penne in a warmed serving bowl. Add the prawns, cover and leave for 5 minutes to warm through.
6 Mix in the pesto sauce and serve sprinkled with extra parsley.

RICH IN Relaxing starches from the penne, zinc from the shrimps, cleansing volatile oils from the basil, calcium from the cheese

three-day detox diet

This three-day plan is pretty low in calories and you will feel hungry from time to time. Don't spoil the effect by cheating. You won't be drinking coffee, and only very weak tea without milk or sugar, so your caffeine intake will come to an abrupt halt. The combination of less food, no coffee and the effects of detoxification will almost certainly cause a headache. Drink masses of water and try to avoid painkillers. The headache is transient and you are going to feel absolutely great by the end of it. You'll also be full of the protective antioxidants you need.

Do the first two days when your workload is at its lightest. To help overcome the hunger pangs, take two teaspoons of the Swiss Herbal Tonic BioStrath Elixir three times a day. If you don't have a juicer, Biotta Organic vegetable juices are salt-free, delicious and available from good health-food stores. Drink at least four pints of fluid – water, weak black tea or herb tea – each day.

This plan will stimulate your metabolism and almost certainly result in three to four pounds weight loss. If necessary you can repeat the detox after two weeks, but you should not do it more than eight times a year and not more than twice in any three-month period.

DAY 1

512 calories, more than your daily needs of potassium, vitamins B_1, B_6, folic acid, niacin, A, C and E: the powerful and protective antioxidants

breakfast

An orange, half a grapefruit, a large slice of melon, a glass of unsalted vegetable juice, a cup of herb tea with honey

midday

A plateful of raw red and yellow peppers, cucumber, tomato, broccoli, cauliflower, celery, carrots, radishes and lots of fresh parsley; add extra-virgin olive oil and lemon juice; a large glass of unsweetened fruit juice

evening meal

Large mixed salad with extra-virgin olive oil and lemon juice: lettuce, tomato, watercress, onion, garlic, beetroot, celeriac, fresh mint and any herbs you like; a large glass of unsweetened fruit juice or unsalted vegetable juice

DAY 2

1,226 calories, more than you need of phosphorus, magnesium, potassium, copper, vitamin B_1, B_6, folic acid, vitamins A, C and E, and a good supply of protein, calcium, fibre, iron and selenium

breakfast

A large glass of hot water, a thick slice of lemon, a dessertspoon of honey; a carton of natural low-fat live yogurt

mid-morning

A large glass of vegetable juice, a handful each of raisins, dried apricots and fresh nuts

midday

A salad of grated carrot, red cabbage, apple with sliced red pepper, tomato, radishes, celery, a sprinkle of sunflower seeds, lemon juice and olive oil; a cup of herb or weak Indian tea with honey, no milk

mid-afternoon

A glass of fruit juice and a banana

evening meal

Any three cooked vegetables (not potatoes) with olive oil, nutmeg and lemon juice, herb tea or weak Indian tea

during the evening

A mixture of dried fruits and unsalted nuts and as much fresh fruit as you like

DAY 3

1,088 calories, more than your day's requirements of fibre, phosphorus, magnesium, potassium, copper, B_1, B_2, niacin, B_6, folic acid, vitamins A, C and E; lots of vitamin B_{12}, calcium and iron

breakfast

Fresh fruit salad of apple, pear, grapes, mango and pineapple, with a carton of live yogurt and a tablespoon of unsweetened muesli; weak tea or herb tea

mid-morning

6 dried apricots; glass of fruit or vegetable juice

midday

Lettuce soup: soften half a chopped onion in a large pan with a little olive oil; add half a shredded iceberg lettuce, stir for a couple of minutes; add 850ml or 1½ pints of vegetable stock, lots of black pepper and simmer for 20 minutes; sprinkle with a large handful of chopped parsley. Enjoy with a chunk of crusty wholemeal bread, no butter; herb or weak Indian tea

mid-afternoon

An apple and a pear

evening meal

Pasta with lettuce pesto: use the rest of the iceberg processed with a handful of pine nuts, a little olive oil, one clove of garlic and a carton of low-fat fromage frais. Tomato, onion and yellow pepper salad; herb or weak Indian tea

Treat your system gently on day four and don't rush straight into your normal eating. It's best to avoid red meat and start with plainly cooked chicken or fish, some starchy foods and plenty of fruit, salads and vegetables. Don't eat dairy products apart from live yogurt until day five.

cleansing feasts

pizza surprise

There's a definite Italian flavour to this menu. Melon is one of the most refreshing and cleansing of fruits. The combination of low-fat goat cheese and cleansing volatile oils in basil are perfect with the pizza, and fruit in any form rounds off the cleansing process.

- Parma ham and melon
- Airing Cupboard Pizza, *see* page 229
- Fruit Terrine, *see* page 228

vegetarian choice

Vegetarian food always has the edge when it comes to cleansing dishes as the digestion of meat leaves a higher residue of waste to be disposed of. The unrefined grain in polenta is rich in digestion-stimulating fibre. And nothing cleanses the palate like a tart sorbet.

- Chilled Avocado Soup, *see* page 222
- Baked Cheese & Herb Polenta, *see* page 226
- Lemon sorbet, preferably homemade

cleansing chicken menu

Raw fish, citrus-fruit juices, simply grilled chicken and circulation-stimulating paprika start the cleansing process in this meal. Again it's rounded off with a light and cleansing fruit dish.

- Trio Carpaccio, *see* page 225
- Hungarian Chicken, *see* page 224
- Cherry Bright, *see* page 227

chickpea treat

All legumes are rich in highly eliminating soluble fibre and hormone-regulating phytoestrogens. Add extra fibre from the wholemeal pitta and cleansing fresh fruit and you have a genuine spring-cleansing meal.

- Selection of dips (hummus, guacamole, etc) with wholemeal pitta bread
- Veg & Chickpea Casserole, *see* page 223
- Fresh fruit salad

prawn power

Powerful ginger, combined with diuretic celery and parsley, detoxing garlic and added zinc and essential fatty acids from the prawns make this meal a detox treat.

- Ginger Cleanser, *see* page 221
- Penne Prawn Pasta, *see* page 230
- Slices of pineapple drizzled with a little runny honey and grilled

bartlett

supercures

supercures for a healthy heart

In the early 1990s, a French researcher reported on the puzzling phenomenon that, although the French eat mountains of runny and very smelly cheese, munch their way through kilos of pâté and foie gras, drink litres of wine and smoke awful cigarettes, they suffer far less heart disease than those of us living in the UK. This study triggered worldwide research into the riddle that has become known as the French Paradox. Professor Jacques Richard found that the French, who habitually eat rich food, drink more wine and smoke more cigarettes, were thirty percent less likely to have heart disease than Brits.

He also discovered that people living in the southwest and Burgundy had a thirty percent lower risk of dying from heart disease than those in the rest of the country, even though they tended to eat and drink their way through more calories. The diet in these regions is much closer to the traditional Mediterranean diet that had been researched as far back as the 1950s and 60s. That's when scientists realized there was something about the Mediterranean lifestyle.

They observed that men in Crete were much less likely to develop heart disease than those in America or the UK. The risk of Greek men dying prematurely was ninety percent less than that of a Brit. When more recent studies showed that men who had already suffered a heart attack, then switched to a Mediterranean diet, cut the chances of a second attack by seventy percent, the French Paradox became even more exciting.

So, what is this strange dilemma and what does it mean to you when you wheel your shopping trolley around the supermarket?

I believe that the answer to the riddle is balance. The French, wherever they live, achieve a much healthier balance of eating than we do. Although they're famous for their cheeses, pâtés and salamis, they tend to consume less red meat. It's also certain that their consumption of heart-damaging animal fats is quite high, yet this is counterbalanced by the fact that they hardly use the ready meals, take-aways and convenience foods that have such high levels of hidden fat.

Even in the Germanic Alsace region, winter salads are made with raw red and white cabbage, turnips and carrots marinated in vinegar and served with a walnut oil dressing – a health treat for any heart. It's extraordinary that just across the Channel from us in the UK, a traditional meat stew for ten is made with beef rump, cured ham, ten each of carrots, turnips and leeks, six onions, four swedes and a whole cabbage. It's served with one giant dumpling – made from buckwheat flour, eggs, 55g (2oz) fat, 115g (4oz) raisins and 115g prunes – which is cooked in the stew. The striking thing about this meal is that it is overflowing with protective antioxidants and, like the whole pattern of French eating, contains massively more vegetables than you'd get with any UK recipe.

the naturopath's view

Naturopaths like me have been advocating the French and Mediterranean styles of eating for a hundred years. Of course in today's commercial world, the red-wine industry quickly jumped on the bandwagon and claimed that all the benefits came from drinking the product of their vineyards – so much so that even the American Health Department allowed red-wine labels to carry a health benefit message. Next came the olive-oil producers; the EC has a vast lake it's desperate to get rid of. They said it had nothing to do with the wine but was all down to the type of oil people consumed.

The truth in fact is far simpler. The French Paradox is not the result of consuming more or less of just one product, but the cumulative benefit of traditional French eating habits. Prevention of heart disease is just one benefit of the French Paradox, but there are many others. The French in general, and those living closer to the Mediterranean in particular, have less bowel cancer, fewer circulatory problems, a lower incidence of osteoporosis, less rheumatic disease and fewer people suffering from eating disorders and food allergies.

France is a large country with strong regional food traditions, but in spite of these variations, the effects of the French Paradox apply throughout the country.

the importance of attitude

The other vital factor that makes the French Paradox and the Mediterranean diet what it is, is attitude. In this country the health police, nutrition fascists and dubious food doctors have made food a dirty word. People are so obsessed with the dangers of food that they've almost come to regard it more as a poison than a nutrient. The French, along with all the Mediterraneans, talk about food, discuss recipes, make enough time to enjoy their meals and savour the glass of wine. Their whole relationship with food revolves around pleasure and enjoyment.

Sadly, there's one Mediterranean exception: Malta. This beautiful island may be the bravest in the world, but thanks to their British heritage and generations of our troops, the Maltese have acquired all our bad eating habits. It's the one place in this sun-drenched sea where heart disease is a major health risk.

So it isn't just the wine or just the sunshine but a complex mixture of all the factors that make up the French Paradox.

paradox shopping

Because they tend to eat seasonally, the French consume a much wider range of foods throughout the year. This is the key to guaranteeing an adequate intake of all the essential nutrients. If you want to enjoy all the benefits of the French Paradox, choose the following foods as you trundle your trolley around your local supermarket.

Red wine Happily, it's a major part of the Paradox. The chemical resveratrol occurs in red grape skins. Although alcohol itself has some benefits, it's this powerful antioxidant that protects your heart and blood vessels. Two glasses daily gives your heart health a boost, and it isn't hard to take regularly. Unsweetened red grape juice is a reasonable alternative if you're a teetotaller.

health advantages of the french diet

- It's lower in saturated fatty acids, the animal fats that are a major contributor to heart disease.

- It's rich in polyunsaturated fatty acids from vegetable oils, which do not cause heart disease.

- It's very rich in mono-unsaturated fatty acids from olive oil, nuts and seeds, which help the body to get rid of cholesterol and protect your heart and arteries.

- It's rich in dietary fibre, which improves digestion and bowel function and protects against some forms of cancer.

- It contains lots of chemicals called polyphenols from red wine, fruits and vegetables, which are protective and anti-ageing antioxidants.

- It contains less red meat and far more fish and shellfish, which means less bad fat, more good fat and more minerals, especially iodine, zinc and selenium.

- The French cook more and use little convenience food. This also helps reduce their fat consumption and has a dramatic effect on keeping their intake of salt at far lower levels than ours.

As much fruit, vegetables and fresh salad as you can carry The French and the Mediterraneans eat around ten times as much as we do. These provide vast amounts of essential vitamin C, betacarotene, folic acid, fibre and the other protective plant chemicals. Eat as much as you like – fresh, cooked, in soups or juiced.

Bread, pasta, rice, beans, lentils, chickpeas, potatoes All are staples in the French housewife's cupboard. Lots of healthy calories, fibre and minerals make these cheap and filling foods essential. Aim at getting around half your total calories from this group.

Olive oil This is the perfect substitute for lard, margarine or butter in nearly all cooking. It's also fabulous to dip your bread in and can be used in baking bread, pastry, cakes, brioche and mashed potato. Olive oil is also rich in vitamin E and heart-protective mono-unsaturated fats, yet contains none of the saturated fat of butter or the equally dangerous transfats (unsaturated fatty acids) that are found in margarines.

Garlic and other fresh herbs The use of herbs in cooking was exported to France by English royal chefs in the Middle Ages as much for medicinal value as flavour. Garlic especially protects the heart, and each herb imparts its own unique health benefit.

Fish All types of fresh fish and shellfish are non-fat sources of proteins, minerals and vitamins. Oily fish, whether fresh or canned, provides the essential omega-3 fats that protect heart and joints and are vital for brain development.

Cheese In spite of it's bad reputation, cheese is a rich source of calcium, which is essential for building strong bones. If you only eat the runny bit in the middle of your Brie or Camembert you get half the fat and all the benefits.

practical tips for healthy eating

- Drink two glasses of red wine a day

- Eat at least four portions a day of fresh vegetables

- Eat at least three portions a day of fresh fruit

- Have between five and eight servings of starchy food a day
  (This does not include biscuits, cakes and puddings)

- Eat three small portions of protein foods daily – mostly fish,
  pulses, cheese, poultry and occasionally red meat

- Use modest amounts of fats and oils – stick to olive, rape-seed,
  safflower – and small amounts of butter

- Don't consume more than 100 calories worth of sweets or
  chocolates daily

- Finally, don't be a fanatic about denying yourself the odd treat
  now and then. Most proverbs and adages have their bases in truth,
  and a little of what you fancy really *does* do you good

supercures for healthy joints

'At your age, what do you expect? It's arthritis.' Doctors often make this diagnosis without any proper physical examination, sometimes even without walking around the desk to look at the suspect joint. The inevitable result is the prescription of nonsteroidal anti-inflammatory drugs (NSAIDs). There are many different types of arthritis, but here we're going to concentrate on straightforward osteoarthritis: a wear-and-tear condition caused by the attrition of living.

The body's weight-bearing joints – ankles, knees, hips and spine – are subject to enormous stresses and strains during an average life. Like any mechanical part, they're likely to wear out. First the cartilage thins, lubricating fluids dry up, and smooth moving surfaces become pitted and roughened. This process can be exacerbated by excessive sports activity, jobs that involve heavy lifting and carrying, or hobbies that apply repetitive strain to selected joints.

Once this damage occurs, the standard procedure is to take NSAIDs until such time as the joint is so bad that replacement surgery is the only option. There's no denying that hip replacement is now highly successful and arguably has brought relief to many people. But what makes me so angry is the medical profession's attitude of inevitability. Little, if any, thought is given to practical ways of slowing the degenerative process or maintaining and improving joint mobility.

NSAIDs relieve arthritis pain, but at a price. The risk of internal bleeding is high, especially in people taking this type of medication continuously for three months or more. The commonly used NSAIDs such as Ibuprofen can cause stomach ulcers and bleeding, which puts 12,000 people a year in hospital and causes 3,000 deaths. The cost of treating these side effects is £250m a year.

natural alternatives to pills

In China, however, ginger has been used for 5,000 years as a pain reliever. Modern science has shown that it works in exactly the same way as many prescribed medicines, even the new generation of anti-inflammatories, but without the side effects. Most of the research has been done with the product

Zinaxin, a ginger-based painkiller, so why isn't the medical profession looking more closely at these natural and safe alternatives? Glucosamine, Seatone (green-lipped mussel extract), and herbal medicines such as Devil's Claw and willow extracts can all be helpful, so if one doesn't work for you, try another.

Cod liver oil has been found to mimic the activity of what are known as Cox-2 inhibitors, the most potent of the modern anti-arthritic drugs. Although less likely to cause side effects than the old NSAIDs, these drugs still produce ulcers and death in some people. Cod liver oil has been used for centuries; it's safe, effective, inexpensive. Why don't doctors use it?

'Rest as much as you can and don't put any strain on the painful joint' is another 'prescription' favoured by the medical profession. Nothing could be worse. Every study has shown that lack of use leads to weak muscles, which result in weaker joints, less mobility and more pain. All arthritic joints should be exercised, the body's muscle strength maintained and, where appropriate, improved. Regular massage, osteopathic treatment and acupuncture can all help to maintain muscle tone and mobility and reduce pain.

the role of diet

Changing your diet will not cure osteoarthritis, but I have seen thousands of patients during my thirty-seven years of practice whose comfort, mobility and well-being were improved through simple dietary care. So reduce your consumption of red meat, cut down the amount of sugars and refined starches and be modest with alcohol – especially all the fortified wines such as port, sherry and Madeira. Go easy on all meat products with high levels of additives and preservatives and keep coffee consumption to no more than two cups a day. Dramatically increase the amount of dark-green leafy vegetables, oily fish and all red, yellow and orange fruits and vegetables. Strawberries are excellent for osteoarthritis. Like apples, pears, and celery, they help eliminate uric acid. Drink at least one and a half litres of water every day.

supercures for hypertension

High blood pressure, or hypertension, is one of the most important factors in the cause of heart disease, the condition that kills, prematurely, more people in the Western world than any other illness. You can reduce the chances of anyone in your family getting it. You can even do things to reduce blood pressure if it is already a problem by making simple changes within your own home.

Blood pressure is a direct measurement of the amount of work actually being done by the heart. The higher the pressure, the more work your heart has to do in order to pump blood all around the body. Throughout daily life, the blood pressure varies considerably, depending on what is needed. Your brain must get a regular supply of 750cc each minute, and this is regardless of what the rest of your body is doing. If your arteries are narrowed, due to hardening, silting up with cholesterol, or constriction by nicotine, caffeine and excess alcohol, then the heart has to pump harder to push the blood around the system, and up goes the blood pressure.

Blood pressure is written as a fraction. The larger number, known as the systolic pressure, is on top; the smaller one, called the diastolic pressure, is on the bottom. The normal reading for a healthy adult is around 120/80, and any readings that exceed 140/90, are an indication that it is time to take some action. The lower figure is the more important, as this shows the minimum pressure that the artery walls have to withstand, all the time. If it is constantly too high, then they will suffer progressive damage, which in turn can produce heart disease, or even strokes.

avoiding high blood pressure

It is at this point that self-help is the first and most important step. Treating high blood pressure with drugs is not a cure for the condition, merely a way of controlling the symptom. This may be a vital step when the pressure is much too high, but you can do things to help, even when medication is unavoidable. Many of my patients have been able to reduce the amount of medicine that they need to take or even cut it out completely. But never change your drug regime without your doctor's advice. If you follow the suggestions for helping to reduce your blood pressure, your own GP will soon see when the readings start to fall and will want to reduce your drug intake.

There are three steps on the road to reduced blood pressure. First, changes to your diet: cutting out foods that will make matters worse, adding those which help and controlling your weight. Second, taking some form of exercise. Third, changing some of the social habits that have a seriously adverse effect on blood pressure. If you have a problem with your blood pressure, do try these simple, and safe ideas. I think that your doctor will be as surprised as you will be pleased, as the figures start to drop within a few short weeks.

dietary changes

The intake of all animal fats must be reduced. Eat less butter, modest amounts of low-fat cheese, use skimmed milk, don't have more than six eggs a week, don't use cream at all. You must avoid all foods with 'hidden' fats, such as sausages, salami, pâté, meat pies, processed meats, most take-away meals, cakes and biscuits made with fat, and all fried foods.

You need to increase your intake of foods which have a positive effect on the circulation and cholesterol level. Oats, beans, apples, pears, garlic, oily fish and wholegrain cereals should all be taken in abundance. Red meats are best cut out of the diet altogether, but poultry cooked without the skin is OK. In my practice, I've found that the best results come by avoiding all animal protein except oily fish.

Too much alcohol, too much tea and coffee will all add to the problems. Caffeine, like nicotine, is a chemical which makes the tiny blood vessels at the ends of the circulatory system close up. Just like putting your thumb over the end of a hose, this increases blood pressure. One, at most two, glasses of wine, small measures of spirits, half pints of ordinary beer may be good for the heart, but several are certainly not.

the salt factor

The ever-increasing amount of salt in the average diet is certainly a major factor in the epidemic of high blood pressure throughout northern Europe, Britain and the US. While not every single person responds to salt in the same way, it's estimated that halving the daily consumption in Britain would save 100,000 lives a year by preventing stroke and heart disease. This fact alone convinces me that a blanket recommendation to reduce salt should be a major factor in all health-education campaigns.

The American Heart Association advises 3.5 to 4g daily; the average consumption in Britain and the US is around 12g. Approximately fifteen percent of our daily intake occurs naturally in the foods we eat, while twenty-five percent is used in cooking or added at the table. All the rest is hidden away in the processed and packaged foods that we buy in the supermarket, eat in the fast-food restaurant, or get in take-away meals. A recent recommendation by British health authorities that manufacturers should halve the amount of salt they use in processed food was rapidly withdrawn; I can only suspect the malign influence of the food-processing industry. For them, salt is a very cheap ingredient that adds flavour to flavourless foods, bulk to expensive ingredients, makes you thirsty so you drink more of their products and acts as a cheap preservative.

Manufacturers often put 'sodium' on food and beverage labels. To find out what that actually means in terms of salt, multiply the amount listed by 2.5. For example, to find out how much salt you get from a slice of bread when the label reads 'sodium – 0.18g per slice':-

0.18 x 2.5 = 0.45g of salt per slice

That's ten percent of your safe daily allowance. And remember that an average bowl of cornflakes is saltier than a bowl of seawater. So make sure you read all food and drink labels before you buy.

supplements

I always think it's a good idea to add some simple supplements to help control blood pressure. The following daily regime could make all the difference to getting your levels back to normal..

- 1 Kwai Garlic tablet
- EPA fish oil, 1000mg twice daily
- 1 Selenium ACE (Wassen)
- 1 Solgar 200 IU vitamin E
- 2 cups of lime-blossom tea

exercise

Any form of aerobic exercise will help in the reduction of high blood pressure. Obviously, the type chosen, and the effort put into it, will depend on the degree of raised pressure, and the general health of any individual. Walking, swimming, cycling or just avoiding the lifts will gradually increase the efficiency of the heart and circulation. A healthier and stronger heart, combined with better circulation, will help to reduce blood pressure. Exercise also has a positive effect on feelings of 'well-being', reduces tension and encourages relaxation.

relaxation

Being able to unwind effectively is most important. Fortunately, learning one of the simple techniques that help is not hard. Relaxation exercises, meditation, yoga and self-hypnosis are all things that produce a good result if you persevere with them. Massage is also a wonderful aid to overcoming stress – it is also pretty good for the giver as well as the receiver – so get one of the many 'DIY' books on the subject and have a go.

supercures for cancer prevention

Alternative medicine has long believed that the right food can protect against cancer. Research scientists around the world are now coming to the same conclusion. But what to eat to stop you getting this terrible disease is something doctors don't tell you.

If I'd been writing this twenty years ago, the majority of scientists, most doctors and many members of the public would have thought that I was totally bananas (which some of them still do). There is general agreement about the role of some foods which cause cancer, including high intakes of animal fat and their link to colon cancer and the relationship between alcohol and cancer at the opposite end of the digestive system. Fifteen years ago, the president of the Royal College of Surgeons said on my radio programme that he believed time would reveal that the cause of most cancers was linked to food, and that their treatment would include appropriate nutrition. It's estimated that up to seventy percent of all deaths from cancer are linked to diet. There's a vast amount of information showing the protective association between plant foods and lower rates of cancers – but it's almost universally ignored by doctors.

diet and cancer: is there a link?

Cancer is the major killer in our society. A doctor only has to mention the word and it strikes horror into your heart, so it must be sensible to take a very close look at anything which may play a part in protecting you from this awful disease. Scientists at the leading edge of cancer research have shown that people eating large amounts of fruits and vegetables have less incidence of cancer than people who don't, yet doctors dither and procrastinate, maintaining that it would be wrong to give blanket dietary advice until they know exactly how, why and even if, these foods have a protective action.

Perhaps you have to be the president of the USA before you get the best advice. In 1984, President Reagan was found to have a polyp in his colon. In March 1985, another was found, and during the summer of '85 he had an operation. By this time Reagan was on a widely publicized anti-cancer diet advised by the American Cancer Society. What was the diet? No red meat, no animal fats, lots of fruit and vegetables, plenty of salads and regular amounts of good cereals – just the sort of diet that the 'totally bananas' alternative practitioners like me had been recommending for half a century. Needless to say, the news of Reagan's diet was spread across our newspapers and TV screens for weeks. But ten years later, little has changed in the doctors' approach to cancer prevention and food.

There are differing opinions among researchers; some believe that food alone is the key to success, while others advocate a combination of food and vitamin pills. Some scientists are not totally enthusiastic but are convinced enough to change their own lifestyles. Others dismiss the idea that it is possible to increase our protection against cancer.

the global evidence

Examining the diets of people who get cancer reveals the astonishing but simple fact that many of them have consistently eaten less fruit and vegetables than those who don't get cancer. Green leafy vegetables, the cabbage family, carrots, broccoli, lettuce, citrus fruits and all other raw fruits are the outstanding contributors towards a cancer-free life. Dr John Potter is a professor of epidemiology (the study of disease in different populations) and head of the Cancer Prevention Research Program at the University of Washington, Seattle, and it's this type of information which has made him a crusader on behalf of better nutrition.

'I think there is fairly strong awareness that diet and cancer are related,' he says, 'but even when doctors in general practice know that this association is fairly widely held, they may not believe it. They know more about things that increase risk than they do about positive things that decrease risk, but today the public is better informed, so that creates some pressure from the bottom upwards on the medical profession. Sadly, like most information, it's more common among the better-educated and the better-paid.

'Unfortunately,' he continues, 'knowing about these links sometimes leads people to think there must be a magic bullet which they interpret as "If only I can take enough of the right pills, I can protect myself against cancer" – and that's probably not true. For some people, taking lots of multivitamin tablets is just a way of making expensive urine – not an alternative to eating the right food. Not all of the beneficial things in fruit and veg are known about yet, let alone added to vitamin pills.'

exploring the dietary link

Most of the information currently available shows that high consumption of fruit and vegetables reduces the risk of cancer by no more than fifty percent, although experts like John Potter think this a very conservative estimate. Of course it's hard to change the eating habits of an entire population, but even if it only halves the risk of cancer, isn't it madness to ignore the evidence? If a drug company produced a pill tomorrow that was guaranteed to reduce cancer risk and equally guaranteed to have not a single adverse side effect, their shareholders would make millions overnight, and we'd all be popping a pill a day. How does that differ from eating more carrots, cabbage or broccoli?

The Hammersmith Hospital in London is a leading centre of excellence for the treatment of cancer and one of its past professors of clinical oncology was Karol Sikora, a serious sceptic about the value of dietary changes. When I spoke with him while he was still at the hospital, Sikora agreed that, in the UK, we have one of the worst records for breast cancer and we eat more fat than any country in the Western world, but he's not convinced by the link between fat in the diet and breast cancer.

'There's no laboratory proof,' he maintains, 'and although there's a hint in the epidemiology, it's not enough to recommend a drastic change in lifestyle to people. All we can say is that we know that lowering animal fat and increasing fibre protects you from a whole range of different disorders, probably including cancer. Are there protective foods like raw vegetables which have cancer protectors in them? The answer is yes, there are, but how significant are they? Whether or not you eat a raw carrot or fresh fruit every day, it's not going to make a big difference. Epidemiological studies have not shown major differences.'

In spite of the fact that in many countries where it's normal to eat far more fresh produce than here in Britain, there are considerably fewer women with breast cancer, Professor Sikora thinks there are too many 'complications' to say it's all due to diet. But would he advise his own family to change the way they eat? 'The answer, personally, is yes,' he admitted, 'but I don't do so much myself. For general health it's better to have a high-fibre, low-fat diet as much as possible and to eat fresh fruit and vegetables every day. But don't think of it as preventing cancer; think of it as making yourself feel better. Think of it also as preventing heart disease, bowel disorder, diverticulitis and a variety of other diseases. Don't think it's going to prevent you getting cancer necessarily.'

the 'replacement' argument

Some of the sceptics explain away the cancer protection of fresh produce by saying that eating more of these foods pushes the baddies like fats and red meat out of the diet. A vehement opponent of this argument and a keen supporter of taking extra vitamins as well is Gladys Block, another professor of epidemiology and human nutrition at the University of California, Berkeley.

'I'm actually willing to be more forthright than most researchers are,' Block says. 'I have almost no doubt at all about the relationship between fruit and vegetables and cancer risk as well as other chronic diseases. I don't say there's a hundred percent chance of anything – including the sun coming up tomorrow – so I reserve a little bit of doubt that it could turn out to be something else. I'm convinced by the combination of epidemiological studies and laboratory studies. The studies are worldwide, covering cultures that have different habits to ours in the US or the UK. For that reason I'm not persuaded by the argument that says "maybe it's not the fruit and vegetables, maybe it's simply that they have a low-fat diet", because in many countries the other side of the coin is not "low meat" but "rice or beans". When you look at countries in Asia, what is the high fruit and veg diet replacing? It's not pushing out meat; it's not pushing out a high-fat diet. Even in those countries where they don't have a high-fat diet anyway, the people who eat more fruits and vegetables have lower incidences of some cancers.

'As I said,' she continues, 'what persuades me is the conjunction of epidemiology and laboratory science because if it were *just* the epidemiology it'd be uncertain; if there were *just* the laboratory science, you'd be uncertain. But they're both pointing to the same thing. There's hundreds or perhaps thousands of test-tube, biochemical research or animal data indicating that oxidation is a real source of damage to lipids and to DNA, and that antioxidants of various sorts can reverse or prevent that damage – can prevent cells from transforming, can prevent oxidants or other carcinogens from leading to cancer.'

what the sceptics eat

Dr Michael Hill is a researcher at the Lady Sobel Gastrointestinal Unit at Wexham Park Hospital in Slough. He's also editor of the *European Journal of Cancer Prevention* and chairman of the European Cancer Prevention Organisation. He's very cynical about the funding for research into cancer prevention. Only five percent of all the money spent on cancer goes into this area, and a sizable chunk to the sexy field of genetics, but by far the largest proportion goes to treatment research, the most profitable area for the drug companies. He claims to be a sceptic when it comes to diet and cancer, but only because he doesn't think that there is enough evidence yet for the experts to be telling people what to do.

There's also the question of outrageous claims made by many scientists during the last twenty years just to get publicity and secure grants for their own research which worry him. In spite of his reservations, however, Dr Hill is quick to take his own medicine.

'There's one area where I actually apply the research to myself,' he confesses. 'I eat a lot of salads and a lot of fruit. And this is the one bit of the diet and cancer story that I think we can really tell the world about. The thing about the fruits and vegetables story is that it applies across the board. It's all cancers. As your standard of living goes up, your tumour moves down in your gut – but you still seem to get it. Given the choice and knowing the odds, I would back a surgeon to cure me of colon cancer much better than stomach cancer.'

To illustrate the difficulties, Hill tells an amusing story of his attempts to persuade his colleagues in the European Cancer Prevention Organisation that one way to reduce cancer would be to eat less fried food, so everyone should be encouraged to throw away their frying pans.

'The Spaniards nearly slaughtered us,' he recalls. 'I hadn't realized that the Spaniards fry anything that doesn't move! But they fry it in olive oil. And as they said, they fry everything; they don't get any of the cancers or heart disease that we were talking about. So why should they throw away their frying pans?

'If my best friend came and actually solicited advice I would say that probably the first thing to do about food is to enjoy it. Because a lot more problems come from angst and worries and general stress than from cancer. Cancer's a disease of old age, isn't it? You can have a horrible time in your thirties, forties and fifties from life in general, which can be alleviated by a good meal, and a bottle of wine, even. If you spend all those years agonizing over your grated carrot and your mung beans, and then get cancer when you're seventy, you're going to be pretty miffed! So, I would say that it's important that they shouldn't just look at cancer; they should look at the whole of disease.

From that point of view, the best thing for them to do is to maintain good body-weight by exercise. I don't think that trying to starve yourself is a good way to get good body-weight; it doesn't work. Going for walks, gardening – whatever you like to do, get as much exercise as you can.

'Secondly, I would say everybody in this country eats between meals. You don't see this in Italy – in the Mediterranean. When I feel hungry between meals, I've started eating fruit instead of chocolate or biscuits or sticky buns. I eat fruit – I like it – so that's easy advice for me to give. I carry a banana around in my briefcase in case I get peckish, because you can't go to a shop and buy a single banana. You can buy a bar of chocolate, you can buy those little packets of three biscuits or a danish pastry, but you can't buy a banana, orange or a piece of fruit. So I carry it with me. I find it a jolly good thing to eat between meals. I enjoy wholemeal bread, I enjoy a high-vegetable, high-fibre diet.'

eating for good health

One thing all the experts agree on is that increasing the total amount of fresh produce cannot possibly cause harm to anyone. They don't all agree that the evidence for cancer protection is strong enough to make blanket recommendations. But it seems foolhardy in the extreme to ignore not only scientists like Gladys Block, Michael Hill and John Potter, but also the accumulated wisdom of all our forebears who survived against all the odds on a diet that was mainly fruit, vegetables, nuts and seeds.

Despite some scientific misgivings then, vegetables and fruit contain an anti-cancer cocktail we abandon at our peril, yet our consumption of fresh produce in the UK is desperately low. One ounce a day of salads and vegetables and two ounces of fresh fruit is the average. Three-quarters of adults don't eat a single piece of citrus fruit, half of them don't eat an apple or a pear and two-thirds don't touch a green vegetable in a week. For maximum cancer protection as well as general health benefits, we should all be aiming at eating a minimum of one pound of fresh produce each day, excluding potatoes. Maximum protection comes from the widest selection, so don't just eat frozen peas.

Everyone knows that fruits, salads and vegetables supply essentials like vitamins and minerals, but even many scientists are unaware of the powerful chemical substances that Nature produces within them. These 'phyto-chemicals' play a major part in the protective action which these foods have against cancers and other diseases. Without these essential nutrients individual cells in the human body are not able to function properly and as a result they can lose their protective mechanisms and may become more susceptible to cancer-causing substances.

The list on the next page shows what foods to eat to help protect you against specific cancers.

Lung cancer Eating plenty of carrots and green leafy vegetables specifically reduces the risk of lung cancer.

Colon cancer All cruciferous vegetables such as cabbage, kale, Brussels sprouts, broccoli, cauliflower, mustard, radish, swede. Chinese cabbage and carrots, are also important.

Rectal cancer There are consistent reports of a lower incidence of rectal cancer in those eating large amounts of all vegetables and fruits.

Upper respiratory/digestive cancers Increased consumption of fruit is linked to a lower risk of cancers of the mouth, pharynx, larynx and oesophagus, and eating more vegetables is also particularly linked to less cancer of the larynx.

Stomach cancer A general increase in fruit consumption and the specific vegetables lettuce, onions, tomatoes, celery and garlic are all associated with a reduced risk of stomach cancer. These benefits are especially seen when large amounts of raw produce are eaten. A high intake of canned fruit and potatoes has been shown by some studies to increase the risk of stomach cancer.

Pancreatic cancer Almost every study of this cancer has shown that eating a variety of vegetables and fruits leads to a lower risk.

Bladder cancer Carrots in particular, but plenty of all other vegetables and fruit seem to protect against this particular cancer.

Cancer of the breast and uterus The results for these 'hormone-dependent' cancers are not quite so closely linked with vegetable and fruit consumption, but there is some evidence of reduction in both types of cancer where fruit and vegetables make up a sizeable proportion of the daily diet.

supercures for food allergies

Real food allergies can be terrifying and life threatening. It takes only 1/20,000th part of a nut to be a potential killer in somebody with a severe nut allergy. People with coeliac disease, an allergy to the gluten which is present in most cereals, can become severely ill just by using a knife that has previously been used to slice a loaf of bread. The same is true with fish and shellfish allergies.

Around thirty percent of the population (rather more women than men) believe they suffer from food allergies. The real truth is that it's less than two percent. The rest are either deluding themselves or being deluded by dubious allergy-testing methods. It's my opinion that food allergies are in fact the new eating disorder as no one's going to argue with you when you go out to dinner, look at the menu and say, 'Bring me a salad. I'm allergic to everything else'.

It seems as if every other woman I meet as a patient or socially has given up wheat and dairy products because they're allergic to them. This is dangerous poppycock; women need the calcium of dairy products and we all need the wonderful energy-giving and protective benefits of wholegrain cereals.

two case studies

I recently saw two women: friends who'd both been for allergy tests and gone onto quite ridiculous diets.

Sally is thirty years old with two children. 'I got red patches on my face, headaches and dry scaly skin on my hands, which all came and went, but seemed worse after eating eggs or drinking lager,' she explained. 'Mary had an electronic allergy test in the health-food shop, so I tried one.

'They said I had candida yeast infection because of too much chocolate and other bad things. According to the machine, I had to avoid mushrooms, yeast extracts, cheese, eggs and yeast and also shouldn't eat bread, curry, curry powder, sugar, alcohol or yogurt. Fruit's okay if washed.'

Her friend Mary is forty-nine and has always been healthy, but after a sudden shock she started getting flushes, palpitations and mood swings.

'At work, I'm the secretary – I do the accounts, make tea, answer phones and run around after thirty men,' she said. 'Some days I'd just stand in the office and couldn't decide what to do. I thought I was going insane and was relieved to be told it was all due to food intolerance when I had an electronic test in the local health shop. I was advised to avoid all corn and dairy products, oranges, cola and anything with glucose syrup or E numbers.'

There is no evidence that this test has any scientific value whatsoever. It worries me that people without accredited qualifications are giving dietary advice which could lead to serious nutritional deficiencies. Food intolerance, especially to wheat and dairy products, isn't uncommon, but the candida story is seldom proved to be real. When it is, it requires specialist treatment – not by someone with an unproven gadget in a shop. With no proper follow-up after the initial advice and no qualified nutritionist or naturopath guiding their eating, Mary and Sally have been left to fend for themselves.

These women's diets are worryingly deficient in essential nutrients, as you can see below by looking at a typical day's intake for each of them.

mary's diet
Breakfast toast with soya spread, black coffee
Mid-morning Ryvita and banana
Lunch jacket potato with soya spread, salad, black tea
Evening pasta, salad, cauliflower, Brussels sprouts, carrots, black tea, Rice Crispies and soya milk

This thousand calories is less than half what she needs, which is why she's not losing weight. Her body thinks there's a famine and has slowed her metabolism. With not enough protein and desperately short of calcium, iron, zinc, selenium, vitamins B_{12} and D, she's almost certainly anaemic and a prime candidate for osteoporosis.

What Mary should do is get more calories from wholemeal bread, rice, more pasta and beans. She needs more fruit, red meat, chickpeas, nuts, seeds and dried fruits to boost missing minerals, and oily fish for vitamin D.

sally's diet
Breakfast two teas with semi-skimmed milk
At work 2 soda-bread rolls, Flora, tea
Lunch jacket potato, mixed salad, tea
Afternoon 2 Ryvita with Flora
Evening oven chips, grilled bacon, salad

Sally is getting just 1,600 calories per day, rather than the 2,000 that she needs. Her diet contains enough protein, but lacks calcium, iron, selenium, vitamins B_2, B_{12}, A and D.

She tolerates semi-skimmed milk in tea, so there's no reason to avoid low-fat natural live yogurt or low-fat soft cheeses to boost calcium. She needs oily fish for vitamin D; tinned sardines have calcium, too. Tinned beans in salad or bean and root vegetable casseroles will add variety, and avoiding bread because it's made with yeast is nonsense. The yeasts used for bread, wine or beer are different from the one that causes thrush, and avoiding the other foods is like telling someone allergic to strawberries not to eat apples because they're both fruit. I've recommended a multivitamin Genesis (available from most chemists and health-food stores), the calcium supplement Porosis D and the antioxidant Selenium-ACE.

The allergy test taken by Sally and Mary is based on the use of something called a 'Vega' machine, developed from techniques of electrical acupuncture in the 1950s. There is only anecdotal evidence that this method of allergy testing works. General medical and scientific opinion is that it's 'magic dressed up as science'. Food allergies are a convenient way of explaining many health problems and there is an army of practitioners who claim to be able to change your life by diagnosing allergies with a variety of highly questionable techniques.

some common bogus 'allergy tests'

pulse diagnosis

This claims to diagnose intolerances and allergies from measuring changes in the patient's pulse rate. The pulse is taken before eating the suspect food and the measurement repeated ten, twenty, forty and sixty minutes after. Any increase or decrease of the pulse rate which exceeds ten beats a minute is claimed to be a sign of allergy. No proper clinical studies have ever proved this to be correct.

dowsing

The ancient art of divining is usually applied to water. Today there are practitioners who use a pendulum that tunes in to energy fields created by the body. The practitioner hangs the pendulum over a particular part of the body or a food and asks the pendulum a question, 'Is this patient allergic to this food?' If the pendulum swings clockwise it means yes; anticlockwise is no. I find it extraordinary that so many members of the public allow themselves to be put on ridiculous diets on the basis of this type of mumbo-jumbo.

hair and blood analysis

These are more examples of bogus allergy testing. A snippet of hair or a spot of blood on a piece of blotting paper are sent to the practitioner who dowses them with a pendulum and – for a substantial fee of course – sends you a list of everything you're allergic to. And there's often a package of expensive medicines and supplements claimed to cure your allergies.

voice diagnosis

There are people who claim to detect allergies simply by speaking to patients on the telephone and 'picking up their vibrational energy'. Again, for a substantial fee, a diagnosis is made, pills and potions prescribed and subsequent phone calls charged by the minute.

biofeedback allergy testing

This theory claims that toxin imbalances reduce the efficiency of the body and can detect allergies that lead to exhaustion and poor health. Sensors are attached to the forehead, wrists and ankles and produce readings which enable the practitioner to diagnose food allergies. Again, there is at present no scientific evidence to support the claims.

applied kinesiology

This technique uses muscle testing to find allergies. The practitioner tests the strength of a large muscle – the thigh, say, or the upper arm – then places a glass phial of the substance to be tested on the patient's belly button and tests the muscle again. If muscle strength is weaker, then the patient is allergic to that substance.

Although this sounds outrageous and there is no clinical evidence, there are in fact a very few highly experienced practitioners who do seem to get reliable results by using this method. It takes extensive training and years of practice to be expert, but many practitioners have no background medical education – whether conventional or complementary – and have only done a weekend course. So beware.

standard medical allergy tests

Even the recognized scientific methods of allergy testing are not always reliable when it comes to food allergies, and even less so when the problem is food intolerance. The traditional patch tests done by scratching the skin and applying extracts from a range of different foods, pollens and other substances will only determine whether your skin is sensitive to that particular substance. Even a violent skin reaction to a food substance doesn't necessarily mean that there will be guaranteed problems when you eat it.

Medical blood tests which measure the way blood cells respond to potential allergens are probably a more reliable indicator of food allergies, but the only certain way of diagnosing food intolerance is the exclusion diet.

The nineteen permissible foods allowed in an exclusion diet are:

Sunflower oil • Trout • Lamb • Venison • Cod • Hake • Plaice • Sole • Salmon • Mackerel • Pears • Kiwi fruit • Sweet potatoes • Carrots • Chinese bean sprouts • Parsnips • Turnips • Swede • Marrow • Courgettes •

You are also supposed to drink at least four pints of still mineral water each day and very weak herb or Chinese green tea without milk.

After two weeks of eating only the foods in the first list, you are allowed to introduce other foods in the following order:

Tap water • Potatoes • Cow's milk • Yeast • Tea • Rye • Butter • Onions • Eggs • Porridge Oats • Coffee • Chocolate • Barley • Citrus fruits • Corn • Cow's cheese • White wine • Shellfish • Natural cows-milk yogurt • Vinegar • Wheat and Nuts

Only try one new food every two days; if there is a reaction, don't try it again for at least a month. Carry on with the list when any symptoms stop. It's important that you keep a careful diary so that you can check on your progress.

supercures for pregnancy

As sperm counts plummet, women's fertility declines and the number of couples unable to conceive rises, ever-growing numbers seek medical help to have the child they long for. These techniques for achieving pregnancy are amazing – but they are not without risk to both mother and child, they're psychologically traumatic and horrendously expensive. To me, it's beyond belief that so few couples are ever asked about their diets or given advice on the simple changes that could resolve their problems before resorting to high-tech methods.

In recent years there's been a growing amount of nutritional advice given to women who are trying to get pregnant or who have achieved their goal. Sadly, with the exception of folic acid, it's all negative advice: don't eat liver, pâté, or liver sausage, soft or raw eggs, or undercooked burgers or chicken; don't eat unpasteurized smelly cheeses; don't drink unpasteurized milk; don't drink alcohol or coffee; don't eat nuts. Of course, this is all extremely important advice, as liver contains huge amounts of vitamin A, too much of which can cause birth defects, and the other foods are a potential source of bacterial infection that can damage the baby or cause miscarriage. But it ignores a much more serious problem, and that is the vast majority of women don't come close to meeting the minimum nutritional requirements for many essential nutrients. It also avoids giving information on the very special protective and nourishing foods necessary for fertility and for a healthy mother and baby at the end.

weight-loss woes

Fifty percent of women with fertility problems have been trying to lose weight on some form of diet during the previous twelve months. Whether it's a 'thousand-calorie' diet, the cabbage soup diet, the Atkins diet, or any other extreme weight-loss regime, the result is poor nutrition. And inadequate nutrition equals failure to conceive. Lack of essential nutrients can have catastrophic effects on the body's ability to reproduce; as overall nutrition becomes inadequate, the reproductive system just switches off. This happens long before there are any obvious symptoms of deficiencies or there is any real threat to the adult. Unfortunately, this hormonal cut-out does not invariably occur, and the resulting pregnancies of malnourished mothers produce low-birthweight babies.

A study by Dr Wendy Doyle and Professor Michael Crawford compared the calorie intake and babies' birthweight in two groups of women: affluent middle-class women from London's wealthy suburb of Hampstead, and much poorer working-class mothers from Hackney in London's East End. The average calorie intake of the Hackney mothers was 1,689 per day, and the average birthweight of their babies was 3,026g. The Hampstead mothers consumed 2,044 calories a day and the average birth weight of their babies was 3,313g. Many of the Hackney babies were well below the 2,500g danger level, at which point the risk of abnormalities increases dramatically. Although there are significant economic differences between the two groups, the working-class mothers spent their food-money very badly: on take-away meals, convenience foods, and little in the way of fresh fruit and vegetables and good carbohydrates.

diet and development

It's not just fertility and prospective mothers that are the result of what they eat, it's their babies, too. Although there is little evidence of gross malnutrition in women in general, subclinical malnutrition – a problem of very small deficiencies, which can have a major effect on fertility – is a matter for serious concern. The nutritional state of women in the three months before conception is the key to high fertility and to the presence or absence of birth defects, as well as the final production of a healthy baby. The diet for fertility must include a wide variety of foods, especially those that are rich in the vitamins, minerals and trace elements which are essential for perfect eggs. Betacarotene and folic acid are extremely important, as they are closely linked to birth defects. Waiting until you know you're pregnant to take folic acid supplements is too late.

Folic acid in particular protects against neural tube defects such as spina bifida and is vital during the earliest weeks of pregnancy. Many women don't know for sure that they've conceived until the first eight to ten weeks have already passed. Supplementation with 400 micrograms of folic acid daily should start three months before planned conception, as well as increasing the consumption of all the dark-green leafy vegetables, beans, peas and low-sugar, low-salt, fortified breakfast cereals.

Carrots, apricots, broccoli, watercress, spinach and sweet potatoes are all rich sources of betacarotene and you should try to eat at least two portions of these each day. Eggs, fish, poultry, beans, wholegrain cereals are all needed for protein. Olive oil, avocados, sweet potatoes, wheatgerm and sunflower seeds are exceptionally rich sources of vitamin E, which is both essential for fertility and one of the most important anti-ageing vitamins. Bananas, white fish and poultry provide the vital vitamin B_6, whereas milk, cheese, beef, yogurt, eggs and chicken will give you riboflavin, for both fertility and pregnancy.

Iron and vitamin B_{12} are also essential. Red meat, sesame seeds, dried fruits like prunes, raisins and apricots, and even tuna are good sources of well-absorbed iron. Vitamin B_{12} is available from poultry, game, eggs, beef and Marmite. A little-known nutrient called rutin is found in buckwheat, which was brought back to England by the crusaders. It protects and strengthens the circulatory system and helps control blood pressure.

Essential fatty acids from oily fish are vital. They are crucial to the development of central nervous tissue and brain cells, which starts at the moment of conception. They're needed on a regular basis before conception and also during pregnancy and breastfeeding. There are some vegetable sources of essential fatty acids, the best of which are flaxseeds and flaxseed oil. Though valuable as a source of most essential fatty acids and the richest of all sources of omega-3, they are not a total replacement for fish oils. Not all people have the necessary enzymes to convert vegetable fats into the equivalent of fish oils.

Ideally, women considering pregnancy, who are pregnant or breastfeeding should take both a fish oil supplement like MorEPA and Barlean's High Lignan Organic Flax Oil for the full spectrum of nutritional benefits. For vegetarians and vegans, Barlean's Flaxseed Oils and FortiFlax ground organic flax seeds are vital.

allergy alert

Finally, we have to address the ever-growing problem of food allergies. It's not unreasonable to protect the planned baby from overexposure to highly allergenic foods like nuts, but the enormous growth of totally bogus allergy testing (see previous chapter) and ill-informed advice from 'nutritional therapists' means that vast numbers of women are cutting whole food groups out of their diets on a long-term basis.

This commonly applies to all dairy products and wheat and other gluten-containing cereals. This is nutritional disaster to women who are trying to conceive and planning pregnancy, as their low calcium intake puts them at severe risk of developing osteoporosis and the lack of wholegrain cereals means they are missing out on extra vitamin E, B vitamins and the essential mineral selenium. Of the twenty percent of women who believe they have this type of food allergy, only two percent have been found to be genuinely allergic when tested with proven diagnostic methods.

eating for conception

Three months of healthy eating is what women need for optimum fertility. If you're trying to conceive, you should avoid chemical pollution and unwanted hormones, growth promoters and antibiotics by choosing organic food wherever possible. As a bonus, it usually has higher levels of nutrients. You should also avoid refined, processed, and ready-made meals wherever possible, as these will all have poorer nutritional value than you can make at home with fresh produce.

Here's the good news. Although your partner should avoid alcohol altogether, there is no evidence to show that a couple of glasses of decent wine will do you anything but good.

the man's role

It's nearly always women who bear the brunt of tests, investigations and treatments when conception becomes a problem. But it's just as often a problem with men that's causing difficulties. For the male half of the fertility equation, the solutions are usually much simpler, extremely cheap to put in place and they can be dramatically effective. However, miracles don't happen overnight.

It takes about twelve weeks for a sperm to develop from its first cell to maturity. During this time, it's very sensitive to damage. You must make sure that your body has a surplus of all the nutrients the sperm needs, as well as taking care to minimize the risk of anything that could cause damage. What follows, therefore, is the essential three-month pre-conception plan for men – the countdown to conception – or 'C-day'.

C-day minus three months

• Stop all alcohol. Forty percent of male infertility may be the result of even modest alcohol consumption. Avoiding the booze is enough to result in conception for fifty percent of men with fertility problems.

• Stop smoking. Smoking is the most common cause of damaged sperm. It can reduce male hormone levels, thus interfering with sperm development and drastically lowering the blood-level of vitamin C: essential for healthy sperm.

• Take supplements. I recommend the following: a daily antioxidant supplement with vitamins A, C and E; MorDHA one capsule morning and evening; Barlean's Organic Fortiflax, 2 tablespoons daily sprinkled on cereals, porridge or stirred into drinks or yogurt.

• Vegetarians should take Barlean's High Lignan Organic Flax Oil, 2 tablespoons daily, in salad dressings, yogurt or juice, or 3 capsules morning and evening.

• Obesity upsets the testosterone/oestrogen balance. Now's the time for a healthy, well-balanced diet and some regular sensible exercise.

• Ditch the tight pants. This means no Y-fronts or tight jeans but boxer shorts and loose trousers. Loose clothing lowers the temperature of the testicles which increases sperm production.

• Get off your bike. Regular cycling on the pointed, hard types of saddle causes damage, increasing fertility problems. Opt for broad, well-padded saddles that point slightly downward (combined with 'sit up and beg' handlebars).

C-day minus two months

• Increase your vitamin C supplement to 500mg daily to reduce the risk of sperm sticking together in bunches – a situation known as 'clumping'.
• Have four oranges, a large glass of OJ or two kiwi fruit daily for vitamin C and protective bioflavonoids.
• Eat at least two portions a day of betacarotene-rich foods: carrots, broccoli, apricots, spinach and other orange or dark-green leafy vegetables and dark-coloured fruits like berries and cherries.
• Drink only bottled water to avoid the risk of female hormones out of the tap. They get into the water from women taking the pill and HRT and this may be a key factor in the fifty percent decline in UK male sperm counts.

C-day minus one month

• Add another 500mg of vitamin C and start eating lots of shellfish and pumpkin seeds. The extra zinc you get is essential for sperm development; each ejaculation contains 5mg – half your daily requirement.
• Eat two avocados a week, olive oil and sunflower and sesame seeds for protective vitamin E. Add a 400mg supplement of E daily.
• Cut out the caffeine – this includes coffee, strong tea and cola drinks. Herb teas, China or weak Indian teas are fine, however.
• Eat organic meat and poultry to avoid the risk of growth hormones.
• Sensible exercise is a great aid to fertility, so keep up the good work, but overdoing it can reduce sperm counts.
• Avoid contact with chemical solvents and garden or agricultural insecticides or pesticides and buy organic produce wherever possible.
• Follow this plan until conception – and beyond, if you can. After all, if you've made these healthy changes to your diet for the last three months, why not stick with them instead of going back to your old bad habits?

supercures for children

In recent years there has been much controversy surrounding the question of hyperactive children. This term doesn't apply to those who are simply naughty, badly behaved or difficult. It applies to children who are impossible. They are disruptive, destructive both to themselves and property, they can be violent and aggressive, they have short attention spans and great difficulty concentrating, they have learning difficulties, they never sit still and they don't sleep.

For years these children were treated exclusively as behaviourally disturbed until, in the late 1960s, Dr Ben Feingold, an allergist working in America, stumbled quite by accident upon a possible chemical cause for hyperactivity. While working on a project connected to flea-bite allergies in children, he devised a special diet which excluded a group of chemicals called salicylates – related to the aspirin family and similar to the substances produced by fleas. A number of children who were extremely allergic to flea bites were put on this diet and Feingold was astounded when many of the parents told him that not only were the children reacting less severely to the flea bites, but their behaviour had improved as well.

testing the dietary link

Feingold then began a large-scale study on hyperactive children who had been institutionalized because they were beyond control. A considerable percentage of the children responded dramatically to the diet, their behaviour changing within days. When they were given a doughnut filled with artificially coloured and flavoured jam to eat, their behaviour deteriorated within hours. What Feingold had established was that many of the chemicals used as artificial food additives were salicylates, and he suggested that it was these very chemicals, together with natural salicylates occurring in some foods, that were the root of the problem for some children.

All children with attention-deficit hyperactivity disorder (ADHD) may be sensitive to some of the chemicals. Among the worst offenders is the yellow colouring tartrazine known as E102, which is widespread in convenience foods and especially in many of the drinks, sweets and biscuits aimed directly at the children's market. Over the last twenty years I've seen dozens of children (and their parents) restored to sanity and sleep by the simple expedient of avoiding food additives. It's worth noting that some of these can also be the trigger for asthmatic attacks, eczema, urticaria and other itches and irritations.

the additive problem

Additional evidence of the links between food additives and ADHD became apparent when I was privileged to spend some time with Dr Stephen J Schoenthaler, professor of criminal justice at California State University – Stanislaus, Turlock, California. He was then working on similar studies with juvenile delinquents, who showed dramatic improvements in behaviour within weeks of being fed an improved diet.

Schoenthaler did many more studies and concluded that a combination of improved diet and simple multivitamin/mineral supplements could change intelligence and behaviour in delinquent youngsters. Penal institutions throughout the US have followed his lead and substituted junk food full of additives for real food, changed high-fat and high-sugar items for healthier options, and introduced supplements. Even some schools in the US have followed suit, starting when the entire New York school system switched to healthier food and saw an almost instant improvement in learning skills, behaviour and achievement.

The most disturbing feature of ADHD is the current vogue for the prescription of the drug Ritalin, which is now believed to be taken by around a million children in the US; twelve percent of boys in the six- to fourteen-year-old age group are now taking this drug. The clinical advice is that this drug should only be used for children who fail to respond to psychotherapy, and the 'special precautions' say it must only be used under the supervision of a specialist in behaviour disorders. I suspect that it is routinely prescribed on the insistence of desperate parents, long before other treatments have been explored and without the specialist supervision advised.

Children are often on this drug for long periods, side effects are common, withdrawal is often difficult. Ritalin is a 'controlled drug', classified with other highly addictive substances. Before you allow your child to limp through life on this artificial crutch of a chemical straightjacket, isn't it worth a few weeks of time and a bit of extra trouble to try dietary changes first?

nutritional therapy for ADHD

Natural treatments do work and the first step should be nutrition, not drugs. Because ADHD may be linked to artificial food colourings, flavourings and additives, the ideal combination is a healthy, additive-free, organic where possible, widely varied diet which includes oily fish, meat, poultry, wholegrain cereals, dairy products, fruit, vegetables and a daily fish oil supplement.

Oily fish are the only source of essential omega-3 and -6 fatty acids, which are critical for normal brain function. Oxford University researcher Dr Alex Richardson is a world authority on the use of fish oils in the treatment of ADHD, dyslexia, dyspraxia and similar problems. Her studies show that sixty to seventy percent of affected children improve significantly with a daily supplement of MorEPA Mini: a pure, highly concentrated fish oil extract for children and teenagers.

Vegetarians and vegans risk depriving their children of essential fats from the moment of conception, as none of the alternative oils are quite the same.

To read some of Dr Richardson's research *see* www.fabresearch.org.

For information on MorEPA, *see* www.healthyandessential.com.

the allergy diet

I've used the following diet for over twenty years. It doesn't work for every child with ADHD, but for many it's like turning a switch and going from darkness to light. Persevere, as you will not achieve any degree of success unless you do it properly, according to the following steps.

1 Keep a diet diary and write down everything your child eats. It's important to keep this diary going even after any improvements have occurred. It's worth keeping a column in the diary for general behaviour and school progress. If the diet is working but there is any sudden deterioration in behaviour, suspect that one or other of the baddies has crept in, either by accident or by cheating.

2 Any fruit or vegetable not on the prohibited list of Group I is allowed unless you suspect that it causes problems.

3 Be a label reader. Reject anything which is not one hundred percent free of artificial additives. Nearly all the permitted foods are available off the supermarket shelf.

4 All children enjoy the occasional sweet treat, but you'll have to make cakes, biscuits, pies, pastries, puddings and even simple sweets at home; there are plenty of recipe books. Make your own ice-cream, too, as fruits, nuts or chocolate may contain additives.

5 The best way to ensure success is to get the whole family following the diet. Would you like to watch while everyone else is eating all the goodies you're not allowed?

The restriction on fresh fruits and the two vegetables can be relaxed after four to six weeks. Only give one new food in any forty-eight hour period so you can spot those that might still present a problem.

Usually, a good response will be obvious within seven to twenty-one days. In some children behavioural improvements may be noticed within two or three days; in others it might take seven weeks. If your child is sensitive to or allergic to these chemicals, then you will see a benefit for all your efforts, so persevere.

Note Severely hyperactive children are frequently prescribed behaviour modifying drugs, and you should never make changes to these without consulting the doctor. Until recently, many children's medicines contained flavourings and colourings which cause the problems. Most are now available without them.

foods to avoid: group one

This is the list of fruits and vegetables that contain natural salicylates. They must be omitted in any and all forms: fresh, frozen, canned, dried, as juice or as an ingredient of prepared foods.

Almonds	Nectarines
Apples	Oranges (grapefruit, lemons and limes are permitted)
Apricots	Peaches
Blackberries	Plums and prunes
Cherries	Raspberries
Cucumbers (pickles)	Strawberries
Currants	Tomatoes/all tomato products
Gooseberries	
Grapes, raisins or products made from grapes	

Try the foods in Group One one at a time for about three or four days. If there's no unfavourable reaction, another item can be added. This procedure is followed until all items are tested and those to which there is no adverse reaction are restored to the diet.

foods to avoid: group two

All foods that contain artificial colour and artificial flavour are prohibited. The following list is meant to serve as a guide for shopping and food preparation. It should be emphasized that this diet is not concerned with food preservatives except for Butylated Hydroxy Toluene (BHT). A child may occasionally show an adverse response to BHT.

All foods that contain artificial colour and artificial flavours are not listed, as such a list is not practical. Do not use any foods that contain these substances. The safest approach is to carefully read the labels. Upon checking in the market, a number of items will be found to contain no artificial colour or flavour.

not permitted	permitted
cereals	
All cereals with artificial colours and flavours	Any cereal without artificial colours or flavours, dry or cooked
All instant-breakfast preparations	
bakery goods	
All manufactured cakes, pastries, sweet rolls, doughnuts, etc.	Any product without artificial colour or flavour, but most bakery items must be homemade
Pie crusts	
frozen baked goods	
All commercial breads except egg bread and wholewheat	
Many packaged baking mixes (unless 100% wholewheat, e.g. Allinsons)	

not permitted	permitted
luncheon meats	
Bologna	All organic meats
Salami	
Frankfurters	
Sausages	
Meat loaf	
Ham, bacon, pork when coloured or flavoured, (usually indicated on the package)	
poultry	
All barbecued types	All (unstuffed) organic poultry
All turkeys with prepared basting called 'self-basting'	
Prepared stuffing	
fish	
Frozen fish fillets that are dyed or flavoured; fish sticks that are dyed or flavoured	All fresh fish
desserts	
Manufactured ice creams, unless the label specifies no synthetic colouring or flavouring; the same applies to sherbet, ices, gelatins, junkets, puddings	Homemade ice cream without artificial colouring or flavouring Gelatins: homemade from pure natural fruit or fruit gelatins, with any permitted juices

not permitted	permitted
desserts, continued	
All powdered puddings	Tapioca
All dessert mixes	Homemade custards and puddings
Flavoured yogurt	Plain yogurt: fresh fruits or juice may be added
sweets	
All manufactured types, hard or soft	Homemade sweets without almonds
beverages	
Cider	Grapefruit juice
Wine	Pineapple juice
Beer	Pear nectar
Diet juices	Guava nectar
Soft drinks	Homemade lemonade/limeade from fresh lemons or limes
All instant breakfast drinks	Milk
All quick-mix powdered drinks	
Tea, hot or cold	
Prepared chocolate milk	
Coffee	
miscellaneous items	
Any margarine containing artificial additives	All cooking oils and fats
Coloured butter	Butter icing, not coloured or flavoured
Mustard	
All mint-flavoured items	

not permitted	permitted

miscellaneous items, continued

not permitted	permitted
Soy sauce if flavoured or coloured	Mustard prepared at home from pure powder and distilled vinegar
Cider vinegar	Jams or jellies made from permitted fruits, not artificially coloured or flavoured
Wine vinegar	
Commercial chocolate syrup	
Barbecue-flavoured potato chips	
Cloves	Honey
Ketchup	Homemade mayonnaise
Chilli sauce	Distilled white vinegar
Coloured cheeses	Homemade chocolate syrup
	All natural (white) cheeses

sundry items

not permitted	permitted
All toothpastes and toothpowder	A salt-and-soda mixture can be used for cleaning teeth
All mouthwashes	
All cough drops	
All throat lozenges	
Antacid tablets	
Perfumes	

supercures for women

Glowing health is every woman's birthright – the health that gives you bags of energy, a positive outlook on life and serenity of mind, that makes you look good because you feel good, that means a clear skin, bright eyes, glossy hair. The health that frees you from all those problems women are conditioned to expect.

This well-woman's eating plan will show you how you can secure the birthright of good health and fortify yourself against physical strain and nervous stress. How you can beef up your natural resistance to infection and disease. How you can kiss goodbye to the traditional woes of womanhood. How you can protect yourself against today's crop of disabling or life-threatening diseases, including arthritis, osteoporosis, cancer and heart disease.

eating for vitality

Vitality means having physical and mental vigour. They can both be yours if you follow the simple rules of vitality eating listed below.

1 Have a mixed diet of as many different foods as possible.

2 Eat regular meals and make sure that you have the time to enjoy and digest them.

3 Eat plenty of fresh fruit, salads and vegetables, particularly the green leafy and yellow ones.

4 Cultivate a taste for wholegrain cereals.

5 Get most of your protein from fish, poultry and pulses, and less from meat, which should be as lean as possible.

6 Have regular but modest amounts of eggs, low-fat cheeses and other dairy products.

7 Use plenty of fresh seeds, sprouted seeds and fresh, unsalted nuts, together with dried fruits. Add them to your meals and eat them as nourishing snacks.

8 Drink plenty of fruit and vegetable juices, lots of water and only sensible quantities of tea, coffee and alcohol.

9 Bread, pasta, rice and potatoes are very healthy. Have plenty of them, but watch what you do to them. Lashings of butter, cream sauces and the chip-pan are not part of this plan.

10 Try to eat one-third of your daily food fresh and raw. For the other two-thirds, get into the kitchen. There is nothing as vital as home-cooked food made from wholesome and nourishing ingredients. It is also a lot less expensive than take-aways, cans and TV dinners.

There is no need to feel guilty about the odd treat. As long as you are sticking to the spirit of this eating plan, you shouldn't become a food freak. There is nothing more boring than someone who takes their own food to a party, wrapped up in a brown paper bag. When your friends all go out, join in, enjoy whatever you eat and have a good time. A little of what you fancy does you good, so there's nothing wrong with an occasional chocolate eclair, doughnut, burger or chips, just so long as they are not your staple diet.

premenstrual syndrome (pms)

PMS is one of the most common forms of extreme stress. It can turn rational women into murderers, the most respectable mother into a shoplifter or the calmest daughter into a screaming dervish. Symptoms may include bloating, mood swings, irrational behaviour, food cravings, weight gain, loss of coordination and generally being accident-prone. This distressing collection of symptoms produces physical, emotional and behavioural changes in millions of women in the few days before the onset of a period. Up to seventy percent of women may suffer, and even those who have mild symptoms will be less efficient at everything they do for one week in every month.

Complementary medicine has believed for a long time that nutrition is the key to overcoming PMS. The general consensus is that a good diet that includes extra zinc and B_6 can work wonders. In 1987, I undertook an enormous research project to test these theories. We looked at the ten most common symptoms of PMS:

1 feeling swollen/ bloated

2 loss of efficiency

3 irritability

4 weight gain

5 lack of concentration

6 tiredness

7 mood swings

8 tension

9 restlessness

10 depression

Sufferers were recruited through a magazine article and my radio programme and 670 women took part, keeping a daily record of their diet and symptoms for four months. The women were divided into four groups. Some were asked to change their diet; some to take a supplement of zinc, magnesium and B_6; others to take a placebo; and the final group to take the real pill *and* change their diets.

At the end of the four-month trial there were improvements in all ten symptoms on a remarkable scale. The women who followed the diet and took the pill (MagnesiumOK supplied by Wassen International) showed improvements ranging from forty-seven to ninety-four percent across the whole range of symptoms. It was also evident that although the pill on its own helped, and the diet on its own helped, the best results came from a combination of the two. The women whose diets were worst to start with took longest to respond, but by the end of four months of better eating they'd caught up with those who ate well in the first place.

the anti-PMS diet

Below are the dietary changes used in the trial. First and most important is to maintain a constant blood-sugar level by not going for long periods without food. You need to eat something at least every three hours. This does not mean eating huge amounts more than normal but spreading out your consumption more evenly to avoid peaks and troughs in blood-sugar levels. The changes aren't hard to follow, and if you suffer from PMS, you should give them a try.

1 Cut down on your tea and coffee consumption. Try not to have more than two or three cups each day. Instead, use herb teas, unsweetened fruit juices, or savoury drinks like Marmite or Vecon. Avoid cola drinks as they contain caffeine.

2 Increase consumption of wholegrain products: wholemeal bread, wholemeal pasta and brown rice. Use oats, barley, nuts, seeds, lentils and beans.

3 Eat more fish (especially sardines, mackerel, tuna and salmon), more poultry and less red meat.

4 Eat a salad each day, and plenty of green and root vegetables.

5 Use less salt. Don't sprinkle it over your food, and put as little as possible in cooking. Avoid salty foods such as crisps, salted nuts, bacon and kippers.

6 Cut down on sugar, especially the 'hidden' sugar in cakes, biscuits, sweets, chocolates and fizzy drinks.

7 Keep alcohol consumption to a minimum.

8 Watch out for 'hidden' fats in meat products, and cut down a bit on all dairy products.

You may have cravings for all the wrong things just before your period. Try to resist, you may feel better if you can.

eating for a healthy menopause

There is no need to dread the onset of the menopause. It is not a disease, nor some abnormality. It is Nature's way of preventing pregnancy when it is no longer a good idea. However, symptoms of the menopause can be unpleasant and distressing. Some may lead to medical problems, and some can be the cause of severe depression. You can improve and control them all. It helps to start your action plan before you reach the critical years, but if you are there now, don't despair. It is still possible to make dramatic changes in the way you feel; all that's needed is a close look at your eating habits.

Below is a list of the most common results of the menopause. The good news is that they can all be improved by what you eat.

Hot Flushes The lower levels of the hormone oestrogen are the main cause. Stress, being very thin, wearing tight-fitting clothes, as well as room temperature can all make things worse. Vitamin E can help a lot. The best sources are cold-pressed vegetable oils, especially wheatgerm, corn, safflower, sunflower, and olive oil, almonds, hazelnuts, sunflower seeds, pine nuts. There are also modest amounts of vitamin E in wholemeal bread, dark-green leafy vegetables and eggs. Make sure that at least three of these are on your daily menu.

Supplements can be a great help, and a large clinical trial in the UK has shown that Confiance, a combination of vitamin E, B vitamins, magnesium, manganese, boron, selenium and chromium, is extremely effective at reducing hot flushes, mood swings, headaches and irritability in the majority of women.

Weight Gain This is a regular anxiety of the menopause. Use all the essential foods of the well-woman supercures (*see* pages 280–1) together with a lot of those at the end of this section to construct the weekly menu. Avoid visible fats as much as you can. Make sure you get some exercise each day. Oats, cooked any way you like, are an aid to weight loss, as they help elimination. They are also a satisfying and filling food.

Headaches Often related to hot flushes, and also to stress and tension that arises at this time. Beetroot is excellent here, but don't forget the leaves and red stems. Use both root and leaf, raw in salads, dressed with sunflower oil, lemon juice and sprinkled with sesame seeds. Beetroot improves the oxygen carrying ability of the blood, contains iron and is a good source of folic acid.

Osteoporosis Don't believe the experts who tell you that it is too late to do anything about your bones once you have reached the menopause. You can still help yourself to better bones. More calcium, magnesium, zinc and vitamin D, sunlight and weight-bearing exercise will all help, so look to your shopping basket. It must contain plenty of spring greens, green, red and yellow peppers, nectarines, or any of the dark-green or yellow fruits or vegetables, chickpeas, pumpkin seeds, sardines and other oily fish, yogurt and low-fat cheese. Eat at least three of these each day. The natural soya extract supplement Estroven is excellent, as the plant oestrogens help combat the loss of your normal hormones. A calcium and vitamin D supplement and two tablespoons of Barlean's organic Forti-Flax are also important.

Skin Problems These are also caused by a drop in oestrogen levels. Vitamins A and E will both help. Eat plenty of the dark-green and yellow vegetables and fruits. Apricots and pumpkins are good. Avocado has a special place here, and you ought to eat two a week. Yogurt used as a skin cream is a good idea, too. A monthly facial scrub using a carton of yogurt mixed with a heaped teaspoon of coarse sea salt is an excellent but gentle exfoliant which removes dead skin.

Depression After hot flushes, this is the commonest problem. Calcium, magnesium, and the amino acid tryptophan will all do you good. Get them from dairy products, spinach, chickpeas, sesame seeds, soya beans, cashew nuts, almonds, wholemeal flour, brown rice, bananas, dried fruits and seafood. B vitamins are vital, and you'll find these in liver, oily fish, wholegrain cereals, eggs, spinach and yeast extracts. You must have at least two of these each day. Exercise stimulates the production of adrenalin, which makes you feel a lot better, so try to make time for physical exertion every day, no matter how low you feel. St John's Wort is an excellent remedy for depression, but it should not be taken with prescribed antidepressant drugs or blood-thinning medication such as Warfarin.

Sexual Difficulties The drop in oestrogen affects the secretions of the vagina and the quality of the tissue in the sexual organs. An active, regular sex life will delay these changes considerably. It is likely that many women will spend their later years alone, since most will survive their husbands. For them, and other single women, it does not matter whether the sexual stimulation is the result of intercourse or masturbation; it's having regular orgasms which counts. The vitamin A and E foods are essential, so make sure you get at least two servings daily from oily fish, liver, apricots, spinach, carrots or other green and yellow veg, vegetable oils, nuts, seeds, eggs and wholegrain cereals. Ginseng is a must here, and for all of the menopausal symptoms. It enhances the action of oestrogens, so making the most of what your body is producing. It also has an oestrogen-like activity of its own. Take some on a daily basis.

Heart Disease Young women have a much lower risk of heart disease than men, for whom it is the commonest cause of premature death. Once the menopause is reached, women are just as likely to suffer this scourge of the western world. Good nutrition now becomes even more vital. Vitamin C is important as it reduces the risk of blood clots, so eat plenty of red, green and yellow peppers, kiwi fruit, oranges and blackcurrants. Onions, garlic, leeks, chives and spring onions are good for reducing cholesterol, as is lecithin from eggs, soya beans and liver. Also eat plenty of other soya products, especially tofu.

Of course, the most important single factor in heart disease is smoking, followed by your choice of parents. Though you can't do anything about the latter, you can give up tobacco, watch your weight, keep physically active, and almost as important as all of these, control your stress levels.

essential foods for the menopause

sesame seeds
Very rich in protein, iron and zinc.

red, green and yellow peppers
These are an excellent source of vitamin C, but the red and yellow ones also provide a good supply of vitamin A.

beetroot
They contain iron and are a good source of folic acid.

oats
A good source of easily digested protein, B-complex vitamins, some vitamin E, calcium, magnesium, potassium and silica.

spring greens
Contain potassium, calcium and iron. A very rich source of vitamins A and C.

chickpeas
A super menopause food as they supply protein, vitamins A, C and some of the B complex. Also calcium, iron, zinc, potassium, magnesium and phosphorus.

nectarines
These supply the essential Vitamin A.

ginseng
This has a powerful tonic and stimulating effect, so is great if you feel a bit down. Take it as a tea in small but regular doses.

soya
Rich in plant isoflavones, the natural hormone alternative. Eat soya in any form: beans, tofu or soya milk.

healing foods

The following list is not meant to be your sole method of diagnosis and treatment of whatever it is that ails you, but it will give you valuable guidelines about foods, drinks, herbs and spices that can all directly affect your health. Here you will find guidance and information about foods, herbs and spices that you should be consuming on a regular basis to help you deal with the problems that may either be the underlying cause or a consequential symptom of any particular condition.

Acne	Cabbage and its many relatives are all rich in sulphur. Fennel stimulates the liver and improves fat digestion. Garlic is a powerful antibacterial.
Anaemia	Chicory is a good source of iron. Watercress contains iron and betacarotene and is highly cancer-preventive. Dates provide iron for vegetarians. Red meat provides the most easily absorbed form of iron.
Anxiety	Basil, camomile, lavender and rosemary contain soothing natural chemicals.
Arthritis	Avoid red meat. For rheumatoid arthritis: reduce dairy products and avoid potatoes, tomatoes, peppers, and aubergines as well as cucumbers. Eat lots of oily fish, ginger and chilli.

Asthma	Onions, leeks and garlic contain powerful natural chemicals which improve breathing and relieve congestion. Avocado is a rich source of vitamin E. Watercress protects the lungs.
Bloating	Celery, parsley are cleansing and diuretic. Mint eases flatulence, improves digestion.
Blood-sugar Problems	Carrots, parsnip, swede, oats and beans all supply good slow-release energy from complex carbohydrates. Dried fruits produce instant energy and slower-release energy from apricot fibre.
Catarrh	Onions, leeks and garlic contain powerful natural chemicals which improve breathing and relieve congestion. Watercress protects the lungs.
Cholesterol	Garlic, chives and oregano all help to eliminate cholesterol. Oats, apples and pears are rich in cholesterol-lowering fibre. Dried beans are good sources of protein, fibre and energy.
Chronic Fatigue Syndrome	Basil, bay, lemon balm and sage improve mood and generate mental energy. Complex carbohydrates, cereals, pulses and root vegetables provide physical energy. Meat, poultry, fish, eggs and other dairy products provide essential protein.

Circulation Problems	Basil, chives, coriander and sorrel help stimulate circulation. Ginger and chilli have similar actions. Oily fish contains omega-3 fatty acids. Nuts and seeds provide vitamin E.
Colds	Garlic, chives and leeks are antibacterial and help clear mucus. Rosemary, sage and thyme are all powerful antibacterials. Pumpkin seeds and shellfish contain zinc to boost the immune system.
Cystitis	Garlic is antibacterial and antifungal. Dandelion leaf tea, celery and parsley are effective diuretics. Cranberry juice keeps the bladder healthy.
Depression	Basil helps ease the anxiety that so often accompanies depression Hops are calmative and improve sleep quality; use as tea. Oats are rich in B vitamins. Bananas, liver and chocolate increase levels of tryptophan, a gentle mood enhancer.
Eczema	Pumpkins, red and yellow peppers, broccoli, and sweet potatoes provide masses of skin-essential betacarotene. Wholegrain cereals contain B vitamins that help reduce stress. Oily fish supply anti-inflammatory essential fatty acids.

Fever	An onion is ideal and effective. Bake one in its skin for 40 minutes, then finely chopped and mixed in equal parts with honey; take a teaspoon every two hours. Teas made from thyme, sage, oregano, marjoram are antibacterial and antiviral. Garlic crushed with ginger and lemon juice is an excellent general fever remedy. Lemon juice and hot water sweetened with honey makes a great fever medicine for children; give two or three cups during the day, and one at bedtime.
Fluid Retention	Parsley is a natural diuretic. Add generously to cooking, as a garnish and in salads. It is also excellent as a tea. Celery is also gently diuretic. Use in juices as well as raw or cooked.
Frigidity	Assuming there are no underlying medical problems, many foods may help: avocados, nuts and seeds for vitamin E, fish and shellfish for iodine, eggs for iron and B vitamins tropical fruit for sexually enhancing enzymes; also coriander, ginger and cayenne.
Gastritis	Sage is astringent and cleansing; drink two cups of sage tea daily. Mint helps settle the stomach; use in cooking; drink as a tea after meals. Cereals such as rice, couscous and oats soothe the digestive tract.

Gastritis, continued	Live yogurt contains beneficial probiotic bacteria to improve digestion.
Hair Problems	Often the result of anaemia or thyroid problems. Can be helped by improving scalp circulation. Eat grated horseradish in a sandwich. Liver and red meat supply enormous amounts of iron and B vitamins to help with stress. Fish and shellfish are good sources of iodine for the thyroid as well as many trace minerals.
Halitosis	Fresh, raw foods like apples, pears, celery and carrots help to protect against gum disease. All citrus fruits supply vitamin C for gum protection. Herbs like fennel, dill, mint and star anise are breath fresheners. Live yogurt maintains good digestion.
Headache	Rosemary, mint and basil are traditional remedies for the relief of stress and its accompanying headaches. Liver provides iron and B vitamins, both of which help to reduce stress. Eating regularly will help keep blood sugar on an even keel and prevent headaches caused by hypoglycaemia.

Heart Disease	Garlic lowers blood pressure and cholesterol as well as reducing the stickiness of the blood; eat at least one whole clove daily in food. Ginger, chilli and curry spices contain phytochemicals to improve circulation. Wholegrain cereals and all dried beans protect the heart by lowering cholesterol. Oily fish is heart-protective.
High Blood Pressure	Garlic lowers blood pressure and cholesterol as well as reducing blood stickiness. Eat at least one whole clove daily in food. A cup of parsley tea two or three times daily is a good diuretic which eliminates excessive fluid, lowering blood pressure.
Impotence	Zinc and selenium are vital. Oysters, pumpkin seeds and Brazil nuts are some of the richest sources. Ginger, chilli, Tabasco sauce, cloves, turmeric and all curry mixtures help improve the peripheral circulation.
Indigestion	A glass of mint tea sweetened with a little honey after each meal and at bedtime will help relieve heartburn. Fennel and anise seeds are excellent remedies; use to make a tea; drink a cup after each meal. Carrots are a traditional remedy for all digestive problems; best eaten puréed.

Infertility	Men should see the advice under impotence. Men and women need an abundance of vitamin E. Eggs, oily fish and shellfish are all good sources of nutrients for female fertility; volatile oils in coriander are important.
Influenza	Lemon balm helps to relieve headaches associated with flu and is antiviral. A mixture of hot mint and ginger tea with honey is a general soother. Turmeric and chilli stimulate circulation and boost recovery. Live yogurt's beneficial probiotic bacteria are mood-boosters. Wholegrain cereals and oats provide B vitamins which help avoid the normal depression following flu. Chicken soup contains soothing compounds.
Insomnia	Lettuce helps induce sleep. Milk, starchy foods, turkey and oily fish provide soporific tryptophans. Nutmeg is mildly hallucinogenic. Lime-blossom tea has a natural relaxant.
Joint Pain	Ginger and chillies relieve pain. Oily fish is anti-inflammatory.
ME	Basil, bay leaf, lemon balm and sage improve mood and generate mental energy, the first step towards recovery. The next **essential is physical energy from**

ME, continued	**complex** carbohydrates, cereals, pulses and root vegetables. Protein from meat, poultry, fish, eggs, dairy products is the final ingredient
Memory Loss	Rosemary is an ancient herbal remedy. Dried fruits and complex carbohydrates provide slow-release sugar. Oily fish and pumpkin seeds supply essential fatty acids for brain function. Garlic reduces cholesterol and improves blood flow to the brain. Sage enhances mental performance. Dried fruits provide quick and slow-release energy.
Menstrual Problems	Liver supplies a rich iron content. Celery and parsley are both gentle diuretics and overcome fluid retention. Oily fish supply the anti-inflammatory effect of fatty acids. Dates provide extra iron. Bananas supply cramp-relieving potassium and PMS-fighting vitamin B6.
Mouth Ulcers	Basil and rosemary supply calming essential oils. Starchy foods like pasta, rice, bread and potatoes provide brain-soothing tryptophan.
Nail Problems	Oysters and pumpkin seeds provide zinc. Olive oil can be rubbed in as a moisturizer.

Neuritis	Wholegrain cereals and red meat supply B vitamins. Oily fish provide essential fatty acids.
Night Sweats (Menopause)	All soy products and beans provide natural plant oestrogens. Bananas contain vitamin B_6.
Osteoporosis	Soya/soya products provide plant oestrogens. Dairy products, beans and peas supply calcium. Oily fish offer vitamin D.
PMS	Liver provides a rich source of iron. Celery and parsley are both gentle diuretics to help overcome fluid retention. Oily fish give anti-inflammatory fatty acids. Dates offer extra iron. Bananas supply cramp-relieving potassium.
Prostate Problems	Oysters and pumpkin seeds supply vital zinc. Brazil nuts provide selenium.
Raynaud's Disease	Ginger, chillies, onions, leeks and garlic to stimulate blood flow and reduce stickiness.
Restless Legs	A common cause of insomnia and fatigue, sometimes the result of iron deficiency. Chicory supplies iron; the bitter flavour is also an excellent appetite stimulant. Watercress contains iron, betacarotene and is highly cancer-preventive.

| Restless Legs, continued | Dates are a good iron source for vegetarians. Red meat provides the most easily absorbed form of iron. |

Restless Legs, continued — Dates are a good iron source for vegetarians. Red meat provides the most easily absorbed form of iron.

Seasonal Affective Disorder (SAD) — Basil helps the anxiety that often accompanies depression; Oats are rich in B vitamins. Bananas, liver and chocolate are helpful in increasing levels of tryptophan, a gentle mood enhancer. These remedies only help to relieve the symptoms of SAD; exposure to daylight or a light box, together with the herbal remedy Hypericum (St John's Wort) should be used for best results.

Shingles — All citrus fruits and buckwheat provide bioflavonoids and vitamin C. Leeks and ginger help relieve pain.

Skin-ageing — Protect your skin with antioxidants by maintaining a regular consumption of prunes, blueberries, garlic, kale, cranberries, strawberries, spinach, avocado and broccoli. Drink 1.5 litres of water daily.

Stress — Basil, camomile, and rosemary all contain soothing natural chemicals. Meat and poultry provide iron and a plentiful supply of B vitamins which help combat the debilitating effects of stress.

Tired all the Time Syndrome	Basil, bay, lemon balm and sage improve the mood and generate mental energy, the first step on the road to recovery. The next essential is physical energy that is derived from complex carbohydrates, cereals, pulses and root vegetables. Protein from fish, meat and dairy products is the final ingredient.
Thyroid Problems	Underactive thyroid may be caused by lack of iodine. Seafish and shellfish are both good sources.
Tonsillitis	Pineapple and pineapple juice supply the healing enzyme bromelain.
Urinary Problems	Parsley, celery and dandelion leaves all contain natural diuretic chemicals. Cranberry juice and berries supply antibacterial protection against infections. Camomile tea contains soothing volatile oils.
Varicose Veins	Porridge, muesli, apples, pears and beans provide soluble fibre to prevent constipation. Wholemeal bread, brown rice and whole-grain cereals give insoluble fibre. Buckwheat provides protective rutin. Citrus fruits, blackcurrants, blueberries supply vitamin C and bioflavonoids. Liver, shellfish, pumpkin seeds, sardines and eggs supply zinc, another vein-protector.

index